The **PROSTATE HEALTH** *Workbook*

DEDICATION

To Rina, Amanda, Rob, Jamie, and Adam

and to

Dick Gross, Dr. James Squadrito, and Dr. David Ellis,
without whom this book might not have had a happy ending;

and to

Muriel Solar, arguably the best medical editor extant, and
Dr. Rachmel Cherner, and Deborah Shain,
for their enlightened and thoughtful comments;

and to

Ruth and Rudi Lea, Richard and Myrna Bloom Marcus, Walter Ferst,
Clarke and Barbara Dunham, Phyllis and Marty Cohen, Elaine and Len Cohen,
and Dr. and Mrs. Frank Rosenberg,
whose friendship would give anyone a reason to live;

and to

the editors and staff at Hunter House, whose encouragement
and support have been a source of joy.

Ordering

Trade bookstores in the U.S. and Canada please contact:

Publishers Group West
1700 Fourth Street, Berkeley CA 94710
Phone: (800) 788-3123   Fax: (510) 528-3444

Hunter House books are available at bulk discounts for textbook course
adoptions; to qualifying community, health-care, and government organizations;
and for special promotions and fund-raising. For details please contact:

Special Sales Department
Hunter House Inc., PO Box 2914, Alameda CA 94501-0914
Phone: (510) 865-5282   Fax: (510) 865-4295
E-mail: ordering@hunterhouse.com

Individuals can order our books from most bookstores, by calling
(800) 266-5592, or from our website at www.hunterhouse.com

The PROSTATE HEALTH *Workbook*

A Practical Guide for the Prostate Patient

NEWTON MALERMAN

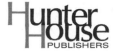

Hunter House PUBLISHERS

Hunter House Inc., Publishers
PO Box 2914
Alameda CA 94501-0914

Library of Congress Cataloging-in-Publication Data

Malerman, Newton.
The prostate health workbook : a practical guide for the prostate patient /
Newton Malerman.—1st ed.
p. cm.
Includes bibliographical references and index.
ISBN 0-89793-364-8 (cloth)—ISBN 0-89793-363-X (pbk.)
1. Prostate—Cancer—Popular works. I. Title.

RC280.P7 M313 2002
616.99'463—dc21   2001051974

Project Credits

Cover Design: Brian Dittmar Graphic Design
Book Design and Production: Jinni Fontana
Developmental and Copy Editor: Kelley Blewster
Proofreader: John David Marion
Indexer: Newton Malerman
Acquisitions Editor: Jeanne Brondino
Associate Editor: Alexandra Mummery
Sales and Marketing Assistant: Earlita K. Chenault
Publicity Manager: Sara Long
Customer Service Manager: Christina Sverdrup
Order Fulfillment: Lakdhon Lama
Administrator: Theresa Nelson
Computer Support: Peter Eichelberger
Publisher: Kiran S. Rana

Printed and Bound by Data Reproductions, Auburn Hills, Michigan

Manufactured in the United States of America

9 8 7 6 5 4 3 2 1   First Edition   02 03 04 05 06

Contents

List of Worksheets. viii

Foreword. ix

Preface. xi

CHAPTER 1 | **How to Use This Book** (and Other Good Advice). 1

CHAPTER 2 | **The Discovery Process** "Is a Digital Exam Something
You Do on Your Computer?". 5
■ Finding a Doctor 8
■ Record of Urologist Appointments 9
■ Record of PSA Tests 12

CHAPTER 3 | **PSA Scores, Biopsies, and the Gleason Scale**
"All Those *Tests!*". 13
"Can You Warn Me Before You Pop Me One?". 13
"How Much Do I Weigh on the Gleason Scale?". 15
■ Biopsy Results 16
■ Questions about Testing (3 copies) 19

CHAPTER 4 | **Keeping Records** "When *Did* I Have My
Tonsils Removed?". 23
■ General Medical History. 25

CHAPTER 5 | **X Rays, Bone Scans, and CT Scans** "Say 'Cheese'". . . . 31
■ Test Records I. 34
■ Preappointment Worksheet 35

CHAPTER 6 | **Diagnosis and Treatment Protocols** "Now That I Have
All the News, What Do I Do with It?". 37
■ Post-Testing Questions. 40
■ Test Records II 41
■ Treatment Option Evaluation. 45

■ *Indicates worksheet*

CHAPTER 7 | **Second Opinions** "Says Who?" 47

  ■ Finding a Cancer-Treatment Facility. 49

  ■ Second-Opinion Questions 50

  ■ Treatment Option Evaluation (Second Opinion) 51

CHAPTER 8 | **Supplementary Therapies** "Quack, Quack?" 53

CHAPTER 9 | **Family, Sex, and the Law** "What Do I Tell My

  Grandkids?". 59

  ■ Family-Issues Worksheet 61

  Blood Issues. 62

  ■ Blood-Donation Appointments 64

  Your Teeth, Your Diet, and Other Issues of General Health 65

  Legal Issues 66

  ■ Living-Will Worksheet 68

  Sex Issues 70

CHAPTER 10 | **Operation Preparations** "You Want to Know *What*?". 71

  ■ Preoperative Exam Checklist 74

  Personal Preoperation Preparations. 75

  Depression 76

  ■ List of Support Groups. 80

CHAPTER 11 | **The Operation** "Do I Have to Shave?" 81

  Post-Op Protocol. 83

CHAPTER 12 | **The Hospital Stay** "Who Are All These People?". 85

  ■ Patient Rights and Responsibilities. 86

  The Hospital Staff 88

  ■ List of Health-Care Providers. 91

  The Recovery Stage: Walking, Eating, and

    Getting Back to Normal 92

  Leaving the Hospital 93

CHAPTER 13 | **Maintenance** "What Is That Strange Thing

  Between My Legs?". 95

CHAPTER 14 | **Incontinence and Impotence** "Am I Destined for Pads
and Viagra?" 99
Incontinence 99
Impotence 102
∎ Sex-Issues Worksheet................................... 105

CHAPTER 15 | **Follow-Up and Clinical Trials** "When Do We
Celebrate?" 107
"But What If...?".. 108
Considering a Clinical Trial? 108
∎ Clinical-Trials Worksheet 111

CHAPTER 16 | **A Final Word**................................. 113

APPENDIX | **Worksheets for Partners** 115
∎ Biopsy Results 117
∎ Questions about Testing (3 copies) 118
∎ Preappointment Worksheet 121
∎ Test Records I.. 122
∎ Post-Testing Questions................................. 123
∎ Test Records II 124
∎ Treatment Option Evaluation........................... 125
∎ Finding a Cancer-Treatment Facility..................... 127
∎ Second-Opinion Questions 128
∎ Treatment Option Evaluation (Second Opinion) 129
∎ Family-Issues Worksheet............................... 131
∎ Blood-Donation Appointments 132
∎ Living-Will Worksheet................................. 133
∎ Preoperative Exam Checklist 134
∎ List of Health-Care Providers.......................... 135

Resources 136

Index.. 141

List of Worksheets

Finding a Doctor   8

Record of Urologist Appointments   9

Record of PSA Tests   12

Biopsy Results   16

Questions about Testing (3 copies)   19

General Medical History   25

Test Records I   34

Preappointment Worksheet   35

Post-Testing Questions   40

Test Records II   41

Treatment Option Evaluation   45

Finding a Cancer-Treatment Facility   49

Second-Opinion Questions   50

Treatment Option Evaluation (Second Opinion)   51

Family-Issues Worksheet   61

Blood-Donation Appointments   64

Living-Will Worksheet   68

Preoperative Exam Checklist   74

List of Support Groups   80

Patient Rights and Responsibilities   86

List of Health-Care Providers   91

Sex-Issues Worksheet 105

Clinical-Trials Worksheet 111

Foreword

Dr. Rachmel Cherner, M.D., F.A.C.P., F.A.C.E.

There is a veritable flood of information available on the prostate gland via radio, television, and the Internet. Although some of this information is accurate, a lot of it is not and tends to inflame anxiety and despair. This workbook provides an excellent exposition on the subject, offering a precise and detailed discussion of prostate cancer and a helpful, positive approach to the handling of the disease.

Cancer of the prostate gland has become one of the most widely discussed and feared conditions in the male population. A form of early prostate cancer termed *microcarcinoma* is to be found in about half of all grown men. Fortunately, for the bulk of the male population, the tumor remains quiescent over a lifetime.

In only a small percentage of individuals does the cancer become activated, aggressively spreading both locally as well as to distant locations. When deposits of prostate-cancer cells are found outside of the prostate, the condition is termed *metastatic*. These metastases may be found in soft tissues such as the lung and the liver and, fairly commonly, in bones.

The diagnosis of prostate carcinoma is made essentially on suspicion, and good physicians will perform routine rectal examinations on their male patients once they reach about age fifty (or younger, in some populations). They will palpate the prostate gland for any suspicious nodules or thickenings. Many times the diagnosis is suspected on the basis of an elevated PSA level (prostatic-specific antigen), a protein material produced by the cancer cells.

Unfortunately, in some patients the diagnosis may be made only when the patient becomes symptomatic, for example, when there is obstruction of the urethra with resulting difficult urination, or when there is bone pain and fracture. However, the disease causes few, if any, symptoms in its early stages.

Newton Malerman, with his intimate knowledge of the subject of prostate health, candidly describes the location and function of the healthy prostate gland and the symptoms of the diseased prostate. He then explores the various treatment choices available to prostate patients and explains the functions of the various members of the health-care team involved in treating prostate cancer.

One of the unique aspects of this book is how the author describes his own personal experience in dealing with prostate cancer. He brings to the discussion a sympathetic and personal viewpoint incorporating emotional as well as scientific factors. The reader of this fine work will be able to clear up any misunderstandings, mistrusts, or misgivings in regard to the details of his own therapy. He will understand the objective of the physicians in his treatment and hopefully will be able to extend full cooperation in curing, or at least controlling, his tumor.

Of extreme value is the inclusion in the back of the book of various sources, publications, and institutional resources where information about prostate cancer can be obtained. Such a resource is invaluable in terms of supplementing the information afforded by the reader's health-care team.

The Prostate Health Workbook represents an admirable, definitive, and valuable reference for every prostate patient.

Preface

Many words have the power to change your life. Hearing the words "You have prostate cancer" will certainly get your attention. If your doctor says those words to you, you have several choices. Some men simply follow the instructions their doctors give them and go blindly into treatment. Others hide their head in the sand and do little or nothing. If you make either of those choices, *The Prostate Health Workbook* is not for you. If, however, you want to learn everything you can about your illness and what to expect, read on. You are a person who wants to do everything possible to survive. You know that knowledge will make it easier for yourself and your loved ones.

When I was diagnosed with prostate cancer, I chose to be proactive. I read two terrific books on the subject. Barbara Rubin and Sandra Haber's book, *Men, Women, and Prostate Cancer,* was extremely helpful. It is sensitively written by two women whose husbands had prostate cancer. The American Cancer Society and the National Comprehensive Cancer Network have produced a booklet called *Prostate Cancer: Treatment Guidelines for Patients*. This slim volume clearly outlined all the alternatives in the early stages of diagnosis and treatment.

I next went to the Internet and downloaded lots of informative data. I talked at great length to three generous men who had had the same illness for some months before I was diagnosed. I joined Us Too, the great prostate website. I got a second opinion. I carefully chose my method of treatment, the doctor who was going to treat me, and the hospital where I would be treated. As a result, I had a fine doctor, and I experienced wonderful nursing and a relatively smooth course of treatment.

Despite all that, I had questions that were rarely touched upon by the medical practitioners and barely evident in the thousands of pages I read. Some of these questions were of a most personal nature, and even my cancer buddies hesitated to talk about such subjects. Therefore, I wrote *The Prostate Health Workbook* as a way to share with other men all the things the professionals *don't* tell us—and about which most of us are probably too embarrassed to ask.

As a prostate patient, you will hear a lot of technical terms that are difficult to understand. I am a businessman and an artist. My job, when I wear either of those hats, is clear, no-nonsense communication. As a layperson, rather than a medical professional, I bring to the writing of this book a firsthand understanding of the plight of the average prostate patient: the need to know what's happening to your body in the face of new, confusing medical jargon. I've been there, and I know that knowledge will help control your anxiety and will certainly increase your odds of survival.

Doctors to whom I've shown this book have invariably reported that it gave them a whole new perspective on the treatment of prostate patients. They rightfully focus on the nuts and bolts of making you better. I focus on how you can fight your disease with the least amount of hassle and discomfort.

The format of this book is unlike any other on the subject. By providing worksheets and checklists, *The Prostate Health Workbook* takes you by the hand and leads you through the complicated and bewildering processes of diagnosis and treatment. A lot will be happening to you during your treatment, and these checklists and worksheets will help you stay focused and organized.

The book also details what you will most likely encounter at each stage of your diagnosis, treatment, and recovery. My greatest comfort lay in knowing ahead of time what to expect. That knowledge helped me keep the pain both minimal and of short duration. It helped me get through the very rough times. It kept me up and fighting. It helped me meet each new challenge with the knowledge that what I faced was just one more hurdle that could be surmounted.

The book's contents are organized to correspond sequentially with the patient's experience, starting with a standard digital rectal exam, through the diagnosis of cancer, to treatment options and recovery. However, don't feel restricted to reading the book in order from beginning to end. If you have a particular concern or worry, feel free to read the specific pages dealing with those issues. Let me forewarn you: I do not approach discussion of these problems indirectly; I write candidly about what you can expect, with no punches pulled. Some of the problems I encountered were unpleasant, and in writing *The Prostate Health Workbook* I haven't minimized the more disagreeable details. I don't want to scare you away, but I want you to be armed with every last bit of information I can pass on to you. A prostate-cancer survivor did just that for me. He kept in touch with me, gave me yardsticks by which to gauge my progress, and provided me with information only available from someone who has lived through the disease. I vowed that I would repay his kindness and persistence by doing the same for others.

This book is written with the hope that it will be just such an important resource for you. Yes, cancer is terrible, but with the help of my wife and friends, I came out of it with a positive outlook and a deeper appreciation of life. In retrospect, there is nothing I experienced that was really horrible or unmanageable. Certainly, there was nothing that even compared with the prospect of dying of cancer. To tell the end of the tale at the beginning of the book, I am now cancer-free, and, in hindsight, the outcome was worth the time and trouble.

One caveat—knowledge in this field is advancing quickly, and information may become quickly out-of-date. Double-check and question everything. Only you and your doctors can decide exactly what is right for you.

Important Note

The material in this book is intended to provide a review of resources and information related to prostate cancer and its treatment. Every effort has been made to provide accurate and dependable information. However, professionals in the field may have differing opinions and change is always taking place. Any of the treatments described herein should be undertaken only under the guidance of a licensed health care practitioner. The author, editors, and publishers cannot be held responsible for any error, omission, professional disagreement, outdated material, or adverse outcomes that derive from use of any of these treatments or information resources in this book, either in a program of self-care or under the care of a licensed practitioner.

CHAPTER 1

How to Use This Book

(and Other Good Advice)

We all live longer today. As a result, most men, as they age, will have prostate problems. It is estimated that over 180,000 men in the United States will be diagnosed with prostate cancer each year, and about 32,000 will die of the disease.

The good news is that prostate cancer is one of the more treatable cancers, especially with proactive, early care. If you have an enlarged prostate, now is the time to start to manage your condition. This book aims to help you do just that. And this chapter aims to help you use this book in the most effective way possible. What follows is practical advice about how to use *The Prostate Health Workbook*, as well as other commonsense pointers about being an active participant in your own health care.

- As the title indicates, this is a workbook. It's designed so that you can easily write in it and tear out pages. Accordingly, extra forms and space are provided. If, however, you feel that tearing a page from a book is sacrilege, take the whole book with you to your doctor's appointments, or photocopy the needed pages.

- Space is provided in many places throughout the book for your own notes and questions. Write down your reactions as you read. Use additional paper if necessary.

- If you are diagnosed with prostate cancer—or any other serious illness—take someone with you to your doctor's appointments. My wife was able to ask much clearer and tougher questions than I was. If you are single, or your spouse or partner is too emotional about what's happening, take a trusted friend or family member.

■ If your doctor will allow it, tape-record your appointments with him or her. In these litigious times, some doctors do not look kindly on this practice. Ask your doctor's permission, and judge his or her reaction when you explain why you want to do so. My first urologist seemed so uncomfortable with the idea that I decided I'd learn more if I *didn't* record the session. I did sit there with my notebook, however, and I asked many questions.

■ Be sure to inform your physician—and all of your other health-care practitioners—of your information comfort level. To be an active participant in your treatment, tell your doctors that you want to know everything they can tell you about your case and that you value their candor. You are entitled to receive a thorough briefing.

■ Before an appointment, make a list of questions to ask the doctor. (See the "Post-Testing Questions" worksheet on page 40 for suggestions.) Leave space to write the answers. Give your doctor a copy of your questions while you talk with him or her. You might even consider faxing a copy before your visit. That way he or she will know how many questions you have and how much time to allow for your visit.

■ If there is information your doctor should have before your appointment, fax or mail the information, along with the date and time of your appointment. Take a copy with you to the appointment in case the original goes astray. Test results, changes in your symptoms, etc., fall into this category. Or, you might elect to deliver this information to the doctor's office in advance of your appointment. Carefully note to whom you delivered it, and ask for a written receipt.

■ During appointments in which you have a second person present, have your partner use the appropriate form, too. Worksheets for partners are provided in the Appendix that begins on page 115.

■ Many technical terms will crop up that you will be uncertain about. When they do, be sure to ask for definitions. If the answer you are given fails to sink in, ask the doctor to repeat the answer or to explain it in a different way. Ask if any brochures or printed information are available on the topic of prostate health. Most people are in shock when diagnosed with cancer or a potentially precancerous condition (such as an enlarged prostate), so your doctor will be accustomed to people asking him to repeat himself.

- When conversing with your doctor, try to restate important conclusions in your own words. Doing so gives the doctor a chance to enlarge on those aspects of your treatment—and also helps to solidify the facts and conclusions in your own mind.

- If you see newspaper articles about issues related to prostate health, insert them into the workbook, noting any questions the clippings prompt. This kind of research often reminds you of symptoms you neglected to report or questions you forgot to ask. Sometimes a new therapy is reported in the media. Your doctor can help you evaluate the efficacy of such a treatment in your case.

- If you have questions, the Resources section starting on page 136 lists books as well as website addresses and other contact information for organizations that will get you started in the right direction. Cross-references to specific chapters within this book are also cited wherever appropriate.

I can tell you from personal experience that if you do take charge of your problem—*starting right now*—not only can you beat this disease, but you can come out of the battle with a greater appreciation of life. Just don't go blindly into treatment of any kind. With a small investment in educating yourself, you can proactively obtain better treatment—and better your odds in the process. You have every reason to expect that if you do so, you'll live many more fruitful years.

Space for Your Notes:

....

....

....

....

....

....

....

....

....

....

....

....

....

....

....

....

....

....

....

....

....

....

....

....

....

....

The Discovery Process

"Is a Digital Exam Something You Do on Your Computer?"

When I reached the ripe old age of fifty, a change occurred in my yearly medical exams. I was told to lie back on the table and cross my right knee over my body. Without fanfare or warning, my internist's gloved and lubricated finger slid into my rectum. Way into my rectum. He probed around a bit and announced that my prostate gland was enlarged (see Figure 1).

The doctor informed me that an enlarged prostate was common in men over fifty. He said there was probably nothing to worry about, but suggested I see a urologist. He recommended several,

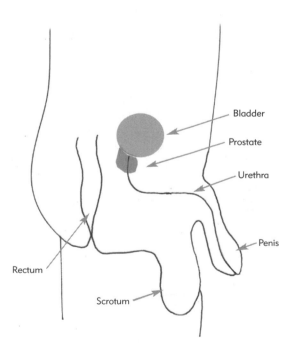

Figure 1. Basic Prostate Anatomy

and I did some research. I picked the head of staff at our large local hospital. He was located close by and had many years of experience with prostate problems. (Resources to aid in your search for a urologist appear on page 8.)

When I visited the urologist, he focused on symptoms I had ignored in the bustle of my everyday life. Yes, I was getting up two or three times a night to urinate. Yes, I experienced periods when I felt a great urgency to urinate and, conversely, times when my flow was weaker than normal. No, I did not have blood in my urine. No, I did not notice any appreciable weight loss. Nor had I experienced unusual back or hip pain.

That history reviewed, it was time for another **digital rectal exam** (the word *digital* comes from the Latin for *finger*). Here, the drill was a bit different. I stood and lowered my pants, bending over the examination table. He handed me a paper towel, which I naively placed on the exam table in front of me. Then he lubricated his gloved finger and inserted it in my rectum. As deeply as the internist's finger had gone in, it was nothing like the urologist's examination. It felt as though this doctor was probing for my Adam's apple. He probed none too gently, pressing hard in several different directions, and seemed to spend forever up there.

I was, frankly, a bit panicked. It didn't hurt, but it was uncomfortable, and it felt as though I was going to ejaculate. This never happened, but during all digital exams thereafter, I placed the paper towel over my penis, just in case. In retrospect, I'm sure that's why he gave me the towel before the exam, and it was convenient to use for cleanup afterward.

I asked him what he was doing. He explained that the back of the prostate, where cancer was likely to develop, could be felt through the rectum wall. He could tell from this rather imprecise exam that mine was quite enlarged (a bad sign) but was relatively smooth (a good sign). He also explained that though prostate cancer was high on the list for male mortality, it was a slow-moving cancer. There were also several other possible diagnoses. My diagnosis at this time was benign prostatic hyperplasia (BPH), subject to the results of a prostate-specific antigen (PSA) test. (See Chapter 3 for more information about the PSA test.)

He said that **benign prostatic hyperplasia**—a fancy term for a noncancerous enlarged prostate—is a condition found in about half of men over fifty. The prostate tends to grow larger as one grows older. The urethra, which carries urine from the bladder, passes through the center of the prostate gland. That's why an enlarged prostate can affect urinary function. I definitely experienced problems with my urinary function, so after I underwent the PSA test to rule out cancer, what was I to do about the enlarged prostate?

There were several alternatives. The most radical treatment is the **transurethral prostatic resection** (TURP). In this surgical procedure, the surgeon inserts an instrument into the urethra through the penis, finds the area that is being constricted by the enlarged prostate, and cuts out the tissue causing the problem. After a few days with a catheter (see Chapter 13), most patients find that the symptoms are gone, or at least greatly reduced.

Another possible treatment is medicine designed to soften and shrink the gland. Proscar is one such drug. In my case, the urologist prescribed a medicine called Cardura, with Flomax as a backup if the Cardura proved ineffective. The Cardura acted to relax the muscles around the urethra to ease my symptoms. In the past, there was no choice but the TURP operation. These drugs have virtually eliminated the need for that procedure.

On my second and third visits, something else happened that helped prepare me for the indignities to come. Our local hospital is a teaching institution, so on these subsequent occasions, another doctor was present who poked around after my urologist was through. As one of these doctors-to-be said, "Same procedure, smaller fingers." She was right. Her exam was much gentler, albeit as thorough. Later, when I chose another urologist to treat me, I found his touch to be gentler and also less embarrassing.

Because of these essential differences in medical practice, I offer the following advice: If you are treated to a rough digital exam, find another urologist. The procedure is not too unpleasant if the doctor has a gentle touch.

If you are just starting to worry about your prostate, I suggest that you begin keeping the records on the pages that follow.

At Your Library

The Official American Board of Medical Specialties Directory of Board Certified Medical Specialists

The Directory of Physicians in the United States

These books list each physician's specialties and subspecialties, his or her affiliations, and where he or she practices.

On the Internet

American Board of Medical Specialties
(800) 776-2378
Website: www.abms.org

The ABMS is the umbrella resource for the twenty-four approved medical-specialty boards. It can tell you what your doctor's specialty is.

The American Medical Association
Website: www.ama-assn.org

This database contains information on the credentials of every licensed doctor.

Other Suggestions

- Ask other patients.

- Ask your general practitioner for information about the specialist.

- Write to the medical school or hospital where the specialist performed his residency.

- Look in the *Index Medicus* to see if your specialist has contributed new ideas to the field. It can be found on the Internet at www.nlm.nih.gov/tsd/serials/lji.html.

Space for Your Notes:

....

....

....

....

....

Date: _____ Doctor: _____

Doctor's comments about the digital rectal exam (DRE):

Was a PSA test ordered? ☐ Yes ☐ No If yes, see "Record of PSA Tests" worksheet on page 12.

Was medicine ordered? ☐ Yes ☐ No Which? _____

Strength: _____ Dosage: _____

Space for Your Notes:

....

....

....

Date: _____ Doctor: _____

Doctor's comments about the digital rectal exam (DRE):

Was a PSA test ordered? ☐ Yes ☐ No If yes, see "Record of PSA Tests" worksheet on page 12.

Was medicine ordered? ☐ Yes ☐ No Which? _____

Strength: _____ Dosage: _____

Space for Your Notes:

....

....

....

Date: _____ Doctor: _____

Doctor's comments about the digital rectal exam (DRE):

Was a PSA test ordered? ☐ Yes ☐ No If yes, see "Record of PSA Tests" worksheet on page 12.

Was medicine ordered? ☐ Yes ☐ No Which? _____

Strength: _____ Dosage: _____

Space for Your Notes:

....

....

....

Date: _____ Doctor: _____

Doctor's comments about the digital rectal exam (DRE):

Was a PSA test ordered? ☐ Yes ☐ No If yes, see "Record of PSA Tests" worksheet on page 12.

Was medicine ordered? ☐ Yes ☐ No Which? _____

Strength: _____ Dosage: _____

Space for Your Notes:

....

....

....

Date: _____ Doctor: _____

Doctor's comments about the digital rectal exam (DRE):

Was a PSA test ordered? ☐ Yes ☐ No If yes, see "Record of PSA Tests" worksheet on page 12.

Was medicine ordered? ☐ Yes ☐ No Which? _____

Strength: _____ Dosage: _____

Space for Your Notes:

....

....

....

Date: _____ Doctor: _____

Doctor's comments about the digital rectal exam (DRE):

Was a PSA test ordered? ☐ Yes ☐ No If yes, see "Record of PSA Tests" worksheet on page 12.

Was medicine ordered? ☐ Yes ☐ No Which? _____

Strength: _____ Dosage: _____

Space for Your Notes:

....

....

....

Date: _____ Doctor: _____

Doctor's comments about the digital rectal exam (DRE):

Was a PSA test ordered? ☐ Yes ☐ No If yes, see "Record of PSA Tests" worksheet on page 12.

Was medicine ordered? ☐ Yes ☐ No Which? _____

Strength: _____ Dosage: _____

Space for Your Notes:

....

....

....

Date: _____ Doctor: _____

Doctor's comments about the digital rectal exam (DRE):

Was a PSA test ordered? ☐ Yes ☐ No If yes, see "Record of PSA Tests" worksheet on page 12.

Was medicine ordered? ☐ Yes ☐ No Which? _____

Strength: _____ Dosage: _____

Space for Your Notes:

....

....

....

Date: _____ Doctor: _____

Doctor's comments about the digital rectal exam (DRE):

Was a PSA test ordered? ☐ Yes ☐ No If yes, see "Record of PSA Tests" worksheet on page 12.

Was medicine ordered? ☐ Yes ☐ No Which? _____

Strength: _____ Dosage: _____

Space for Your Notes:

....

....

....

(See Chapter 3 for an explanation of the PSA test.)

Date	Ordered by	Where performed	PSA Score
_____	_____	_____	_____
_____	_____	_____	_____
_____	_____	_____	_____
_____	_____	_____	_____
_____	_____	_____	_____
_____	_____	_____	_____
_____	_____	_____	_____
_____	_____	_____	_____
_____	_____	_____	_____
_____	_____	_____	_____
_____	_____	_____	_____
_____	_____	_____	_____
_____	_____	_____	_____
_____	_____	_____	_____
_____	_____	_____	_____
_____	_____	_____	_____
_____	_____	_____	_____
_____	_____	_____	_____
_____	_____	_____	_____

Space for Your Notes:

....

....

....

....

....

....

PSA Scores, Biopsies, and the Gleason Scale

"All Those *Tests!*"

"CAN YOU WARN ME BEFORE YOU POP ME ONE?"

Once I was diagnosed with an enlarged prostate, every six months or so for the next several years I went for regular **prostate-specific antigen** (PSA) tests.

When cancer cells are present, the body produces a protein (antigen) that can induce an immune response in the body. If prostate cancer is present, the antigens will also be present. This test finds the antigen that is specific to the prostate cancer. The test results are measured in nanograms per milliliter (ng/ml). Results under 4 are considered normal, since ejaculation, infection, and prostatitis sometimes elevate the results. Results over 10 are considered to be high indicators.

It took about a week each time for the results to get to the urologist, so an office visit followed, as did another digital exam. After several years of regular testing, one day my PSA score tested at an elevated 6.3. During the digital examination that followed, the doctor also felt some hard spots on one quadrant of my prostate. He believed that a biopsy was in order and scheduled one for the following week.

I was given pretest instructions that included taking an enema the night before the biopsy and another one several hours before it. Every doctor observes his own protocol for this procedure, so what your doctor asks you to do may be different from what mine requested, but do follow your doctor's orders. If you are not sure why he's ordering certain things or what exactly he means, *ask!* This is a good time to start taking a partner or trusted friend with you to all your appointments. When you are under stress, it becomes more difficult to listen accurately, so another set of ears is helpful (you might want to review the list of pointers in Chapter 1).

My biopsy was done in the doctor's office. I donned a hospital gown, conveniently open in back. The room had a strange-looking TV set, which I later learned was an ultrasound machine.

I was told to lie on my left side, with my right knee pulled up to my chest. The doctor then inserted a probe into my rectum. The probe is a tube, rounded at the end, and a bit fatter than a pencil. The probe sends out ultrasound waves that create a picture of your prostate on the screen. The doctor can generate a hard copy of the images if he wants a permanent record. The machine is also programmed to give the doctor vital measurements, such as the size of the prostate gland.

Under today's system of managed care, the examination frequently involves two parts. In the first, the doctor merely looks ultrasonically at the gland. If there is reason to suspect a problem, he will proceed with the biopsy. If not, he discontinues the procedure. If you want the peace of mind of a biopsy no matter what the doctor sees on the ultrasound, you may have to pay for it. Check this out with your doctor ahead of time.

In my case, the ultrasound image showed that, indeed, my prostate was quite enlarged, so the doctor announced that he would proceed with the biopsy. He told me I would feel "a little pinch."

POP!... Pinch! Frankly, the pinch wasn't bothersome, but the unexpected POP made me jump. (You are now forewarned as to what will happen.) Ask your doctor to please warn you before he takes a sample. There is hardly any pain involved in this procedure when you know what to expect. It's not something I came to enjoy, but the mild discomfort was worth the certain knowledge gained by the procedure.

During the biopsy, the doctor removes a tiny bit of the gland with each pinch. He charts the position of the sample and then sends it off to the pathology lab. You are then on nervous alert until the results come back. The test will tell two things. First, it will tell if there is cancer. Second, it will rate the virulence of the cancer cells that may be present, and it will assess the probability of the cancer's spreading.

Blood will appear in both your stool and your urine for a while after the biopsy. Your semen will also be bloody for a week or two, so if you don't normally use a condom during intercourse, use one for a while. You may also feel sore in the area for a few days, and you may be prescribed an antibiotic.

When I called in for my first biopsy results, I asked the doctor, "How are you?" "I'm fine," he said, "and, thank God, so are you.

The hard spots turned out to be stones. We'll just monitor you from time to time. See you in six months."

If you are lucky enough to receive a negative biopsy report, as I did that first time, you're home free. Periodic examinations will monitor your prostate problems.

"HOW MUCH DO I WEIGH ON THE GLEASON SCALE?"

So we continued with the semiannual PSA-testing schedule. Then, once again, several years later, my PSA showed up as elevated. This time it was a 10. This called for a second biopsy, which again proved negative. The next PSA result was an 8.5. I had dropped a point and a half. I am telling you about these variations so you will have something against which to compare your own results. Don't let an unexpected result spook you. Let your doctor be your guide.

After a few more years, my PSA went up to a 10.5. This occasioned another biopsy, during which the doctor took samples at random from a section of the prostate that was *not* suspect. Two of those samples turned up tumors. My biopsy had come back positive, with a Gleason-scale score of 6. After some fifteen years of watching my prostate, I was diagnosed with prostate cancer.

The **Gleason scale** is named for Dr. Gleason, a pathologist from the University of Minnesota who set up a scale by which tumors could be evaluated as to their aggressiveness. When the pathologist looks at the samples of the prostate taken during the biopsy, two cells are evaluated. Each cell ranges from 1 to 5 on this scale. If the cells are normal, or just slightly irregular, a Gleason score of 1 is assigned to each cell. Greater irregularity and size inconsistency will earn a 2. Highly developed cancerous cells earn a 5. Adding the two scores together ranks the volatility of the tumor between 2 and 10, with 10 indicating that the tumor is most likely to progress rapidly (see Figure 2).

The results of your biopsies are obviously of great importance. The following worksheets will help you chart your results. Record your doctor's comments in as much detail as you can remember.

Figure 2. Gleason Scale Criteria

  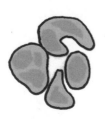 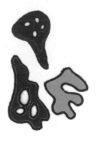 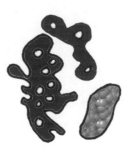

1   2   3   4   5

Date   **Where performed**   **Doctor**   **Results (Gleason Score)**

_____   _____   _____   _____

Doctor's comments:

_____

_____

Space for Your Notes:

....

....

Date   **Where performed**   **Doctor**   **Results (Gleason Score)**

_____   _____   _____   _____

Doctor's comments:

_____

_____

Space for Your Notes:

....

....

Date   **Where performed**   **Doctor**   **Results (Gleason Score)**

_____   _____   _____   _____

Doctor's comments:

_____

_____

Space for Your Notes:

....

....

Date   **Where performed**   **Doctor**   **Results (Gleason Score)**

_____ _____ _____ _____

Doctor's comments:

_____

_____

Space for Your Notes:

....

....

Date   **Where performed**   **Doctor**   **Results (Gleason Score)**

_____ _____ _____ _____

Doctor's comments:

_____

_____

Space for Your Notes:

....

....

Date   **Where performed**   **Doctor**   **Results (Gleason Score)**

_____ _____ _____ _____

Doctor's comments:

_____

_____

Space for Your Notes:

....

....

I was by this time sixty-nine years old, a lucky thing as it turned out. If your Gleason score is under 5, and/or if you are age seventy or older, the recommendation is for "watchful waiting." This is also true if you have other medical conditions of a serious nature.

The philosophy behind watchful waiting is that prostate cancer is so slow-moving that patients over seventy will probably die from something other than the cancer. Watchful waiting means you will undergo PSAs and digital exams on a regular basis to monitor your progress. Another protocol recommended under such conditions is hormone therapy to slow or stop the progress of the cancer. Hormone therapy decreases the level of testosterone in the body. Because prostate cancer needs testosterone to grow, this slows the development of the cancer and buys you time. Few other measures besides hormone therapy are indicated. (More information on hormone treatment and other therapies appears in later chapters.)

Since I was under the magic age and also high on the Gleason scale, the doctor ordered several tests to see if the cancer had spread to other parts of my body or was self-contained in the prostate. The tests called for in such a case might include a bone scan, a chest X ray, and a CT scan (also known as a CAT scan). Suggested questions you may want to ask your doctor about these tests appear on the next worksheet. Three copies are provided—one for each test you are likely to undergo.

Don't expect to get all of the answers to these questions from your urologist alone. His nurse will probably discuss the necessary preparations with you and will schedule your appointments. Some of the answers will also be filled in as you do your own research.

What is the name of this test? _____

What is the purpose of this test? _____

_____

Is the test necessary? ☐ Yes ☐ No

Where do I take the test? _____

How long will it take? _____

Will I have to stay overnight? ☐ Yes ☐ No

Will I be able to drive myself home safely after the test? ☐ Yes ☐ No

Are there any side effects from the test? ☐ Yes ☐ No

_____

Is there any medication I must take before the test? ☐ Yes ☐ No

_____

Is there any other preparation before the test? ☐ Yes ☐ No Must I fast? ☐ Yes ☐ No

_____

Is there any pain involved in this procedure, and, if so, can I take medication for it? ☐ Yes ☐ No

_____

Would I take the pain medication before the test, or after? _____

When and how do I get the results of the test? _____

_____

Where do I get physical possession of my X rays and plates from any testing? _____

_____

What is the name of this test? _____

What is the purpose of this test? _____

_____

Is the test necessary? ☐ Yes ☐ No

Where do I take the test? _____

How long will it take? _____

Will I have to stay overnight? ☐ Yes ☐ No

Will I be able to drive myself home safely after the test? ☐ Yes ☐ No

Are there any side effects from the test? ☐ Yes ☐ No

_____

Is there any medication I must take before the test? ☐ Yes ☐ No

_____

Is there any other preparation before the test? ☐ Yes ☐ No Must I fast? ☐ Yes ☐ No

_____

Is there any pain involved in this procedure, and, if so, can I take medication for it? ☐ Yes ☐ No

_____

Would I take the pain medication before the test, or after? _____

When and how do I get the results of the test? _____

_____

Where do I get physical possession of my X rays and plates from any testing? _____

_____

What is the name of this test? _____

What is the purpose of this test? _____

_____

Is the test necessary? ☐ Yes ☐ No

Where do I take the test? _____

How long will it take? _____

Will I have to stay overnight? ☐ Yes ☐ No

Will I be able to drive myself home safely after the test? ☐ Yes ☐ No

Are there any side effects from the test? ☐ Yes ☐ No

_____

Is there any medication I must take before the test? ☐ Yes ☐ No

_____

Is there any other preparation before the test? ☐ Yes ☐ No Must I fast? ☐ Yes ☐ No

_____

Is there any pain involved in this procedure, and, if so, can I take medication for it? ☐ Yes ☐ No

_____

Would I take the pain medication before the test, or after? _____

When and how do I get the results of the test? _____

_____

Where do I get physical possession of my X rays and plates from any testing? _____

_____

Space for Your Notes:

CHAPTER 4

Keeping Records

"When *Did* I Have My Tonsils Removed?"

Before we discuss the tests you will undergo, let's pause and prepare for the hectic days ahead.

Your life will get quite complicated from here on, and possibly confusing as well. Your brain will be spinning with numbers, grades, protocols, and names. You will be forced to make serious decisions under an overload of emotions. Follow the advice given in Chapter 1 and keep good records. Years after the fact, it's easy to forget when exactly it was that you underwent a major medical procedure—especially if you're sitting in some doctor's office with a stack of blank forms to complete; at that moment, you can't call anyone to find out just when you had your tonsils out. That's why it's important to write down everything beforehand.

The detailed "General Medical History" worksheet provided on pages 25–29 aims to simplify the somewhat daunting task of record keeping. The questionnaire is designed to summarize your general medical history, so you can have the information at your fingertips when the time comes to fill out forms required by doctors and others. Completing this worksheet and taking it with you to each of your appointments may save much time for you and your physicians.

It bears repeating that the purpose of this book is to make you an assertive participant in your own treatment. Physicians are trained to be "take-charge" individuals, but they sometimes forget which end of the gloved finger they're on. It is, after all, your body—and your life. The exercises and techniques contained herein will empower you to take an active role in your treatment. Psychologically, the worst thing about having cancer is the feeling of loss of control. By following these proactive steps, you will be taking positive action in the fight against your disease, and consequently, you will feel less vulnerable. You will most assuredly get better treatment, and you will feel empowered knowing what to expect and what you can do about it.

A final point: Your main job for the next several months is to focus on the many helpful things you can do for yourself. This is a good time to seek out fellow prostate-cancer patients. Those who have gone through the process already will be able to supply emotional and informational support that you'll find comforting. If you have difficulty establishing a network, a "List of Support Groups" worksheet appears on page 80.

You should now take the time to complete the following worksheet, before you get too busy or concerned with other matters.

You will soon be completing many forms. Each of your doctors, the testing facilities, and the hospital will require much of the information requested in this worksheet. You'll be surprised at how much you've forgotten about your medical history when you're sitting in an office somewhere. Filling out this questionnaire in the leisure of your home or office will save you a lot of stress and paper shuffling later. Make photocopies to take with you to your appointments.

Your full name:_____

Address: _____

City _____ State: _____ Zip: _____

Home phone: _____ Fax: _____

Mobile phone: _____ Social Security #: _____

E-mail:_____

Birthday (month/day/year): _____

Company name: _____

Address: _____

City:_____ State: _____ Zip: _____

Business phone:_____ Extension #: _____

EMERGENCY CONTACT:

Full name: _____

Address: _____

City:_____ State: _____ Zip: _____

Home phone: _____ Business phone: _____

Relationship to you:_____

ALTERNATIVE EMERGENCY CONTACT:

Full name: _____

Address: _____

City:_____ State: _____ Zip: _____

Home phone: _____ Business phone: _____

Relationship to you:_____

INSURANCE DATA (take all insurance cards with you):

Primary insurer: _____

Name of insured: _____

Social Security # of insured: _____

Policy #: _____ Group #: _____

Insured (membership) #: _____

Secondary insurer: _____

Name of insured: _____

SS# of insured if different from above: _____

Policy #: _____ Group #: _____

Insured (membership) #: _____

PREVIOUS CONDITIONS:

List all previous medical conditions that apply (be sure to include all previous surgeries), including when the problem was diagnosed, how it was treated, and by whom. Use additional sheets of paper if necessary.

Problem	When diagnosed	How treated	Doctor	Comments
Asthma	_____	_____	_____	_____
Heart	_____	_____	_____	_____
Vascular	_____	_____	_____	_____
Diabetes	_____	_____	_____	_____
High blood pressure	_____	_____	_____	_____
Cancer	_____	_____	_____	_____
Digestive	_____	_____	_____	_____
Other (list below)	_____	_____	_____	_____
_____	_____	_____	_____	_____
_____	_____	_____	_____	_____
_____	_____	_____	_____	_____
_____	_____	_____	_____	_____
Elevated PSA	_____	_____	_____	_____
Biopsy	_____	_____	_____	_____

MEDICAL DATA:

Prescription medications:

Medicine	Strength (e.g., 50 mg)	Dosage (e.g., twice daily)	Taken for (condition)	Since when

Over-the-counter medications (e.g., aspirin, Tylenol, herbal supplements, cold remedies):

Medicine	Strength (e.g., 50 mg)	Dosage (e.g., twice daily)	Taken for (condition)	Since when

VITAMINS/MINERALS/OTHER SUPPLEMENTS:

List contents and strength or RDA percentage from the label of each supplement. For multivitamin supplements, list each ingredient separately on a line in the chart.

Product (brand) name:_____   Product (brand) name: _____

Dosage (e.g., twice daily): _____   Dosage (e.g., twice daily): _____

Ingredient (e.g., iron)	Strength (e.g., 18 mg or 100% RDA)	Ingredient (e.g., iron)	Strength (e.g., 18 mg or 100% RDA)

ALLERGIES:

List your allergies and your symptoms. Be specific. If you need more space in which to write, use the next page.

Allergy	Symptoms	Treatment

Foods (list which ones):

_____   _____   _____

_____   _____   _____

_____   _____   _____

_____   _____   _____

_____   _____   _____

_____   _____   _____

Penicillin _____   _____   _____

Other antibiotics (list which ones):

_____   _____   _____

_____   _____   _____

Dust _____   _____   _____

Pollen _____   _____   _____

Other substances (list which ones):

_____   _____   _____

_____   _____   _____

Other medications (list which ones):

_____   _____   _____

_____   _____   _____

Do you smoke? ☐ Yes ☐ No What? _____ How much? _____

Do you drink alcohol? ☐ Yes ☐ No What? _____ How much? _____

Do you exercise? ☐ Yes ☐ No How? _____

   How often and how much? _____

Other lifestyle issues you need to discuss: _____

_____

_____

Space for Your Notes:

....
....
....
....
....
....
....
....
....
....
....
....
....
....
....
....
....
....
....
....
....
....
....
....
....
....
....
....

CHAPTER 5

X Rays, Bone Scans, and CT Scans

"Say 'Cheese'"

The next step involves undergoing the required tests to see if the cancer has spread. Though my doctor told me there was no hurry to have the tests, I wanted to increase my chances as much as possible. I therefore took the tests as soon as I could and always followed my doctor's instructions to the letter.

There are two seemingly contrary pieces of advice I can give you at this point. First, use your questions carefully. Don't waste them on people who can't give you an authoritative answer. For example, don't ask the person drawing blood about the possible outcomes of the tests. He or she is not qualified to give you an answer, although he or she may respond to your question in an authoritative manner. Don't ask the technician giving you an X ray or CT scan what he or she sees. Only a doctor can interpret the images, and only a physician conversant with your case can apply what's on the plates to meaningful information relevant to you.

The second piece of advice may seem contradictory to the above. Rely on the nurse. Often the doctor will have a nurse on staff who fields most of the routine questions. In both the doctor's office and at the hospital, find this person. These highly competent professionals can more easily answer 95 percent of your questions than your busy physician. If they don't know the answer, they can get to the doctor more efficiently than you can, and they will call you back. (Be sure you are talking to a registered nurse and not a technician or a receptionist.)

In my case, the first order of business was a chest X ray. It is rare for prostate cancer to involve the lungs, but since I had not had a chest X ray in more than a year, my doctor ordered one. Of more serious import—and much more of an inconvenience—were the CT scan (or CAT scan) and bone scan.

CT stands for **computed tomography.** When I showed up for the procedure, I was given two bottles of cold liquid. If you like the taste of milk of magnesia (with the addition of a minty flavor), you'll love this stuff. You drink one pint first, then you drink a second one an hour later, so bring a book to read. I was then strapped lightly onto a hard table. If you find the table uncomfortable, ask for a pillow. If you get cold, ask for a blanket. You'll be there a while.

Next, the table you're lying on slides into the CT machine. The opening I went through was a bit wider than my corpulent bod, but not by much. If you suffer from claustrophobia, I recommend paying a visit to your friendly hypnotist or getting a prescription for a sedative before the procedure. Some CT machines are built with wider apertures, so if claustrophobia is a problem for you, call around or get a referral from your doctor to have your test done using one of these special machines. Your insurance carrier might also be able to direct you to a CT provider with one of these machines.

When the CT machine is turned on, it whirs quietly. Then it almost imperceptibly starts to move, scanning you from head to toe to produce a series of cross-sectional images of your body. You're directed not to move. Otherwise, from time to time the technician may give you instructions. Generally, it is a boring but painless procedure that lasts half an hour or so. The resulting images are quite fascinating. In the not too distant past, a surgeon would have had to perform exploratory surgery to get the information now available through this noninvasive procedure.

My **bone scan** took place in the hospital's department of nuclear medicine. I was given an injection of a harmless radioactive dye and was sent home while the stuff filtered into my bones. Four or five hours later, another humming machine traveled over my body to give me a head-to-toe scan. The plates from this procedure look pretty weird, like something you'd see at Halloween. They show every bone in the body.

None of my tests indicated that the cancer had spread. It seemed wholly confined to my prostate ("inside the envelope" or "inside the capsule"). The most likely site for the disease to spread to is the lymph nodes, and in my case these seemed clear, although during surgery they were removed anyway—a wise precaution.

I have one strong word of advice. Insist during all of these procedures that you want to retain possession of the films. If asked why, say that you need them for a second opinion. You are paying for them, either out of pocket or via insurance, and you are entitled to them. This may necessitate some running around to collect them all. Use the "Test-Records I" worksheet on page 34 to organize this process. Make sure that when you pick up the pictures, the reports are included. If possible, your growing file should also include the ultrasounds and pathologist's reports from your biopsy.

In the event that a hospital or lab refuses to release the originals, and your doctor or second consult needs them, inquire about obtaining a copy. This can be an expensive procedure, but in all likelihood you will not face this problem. A direct request from your physician will usually get the material released.

You will now have several different images of your body. The standard X ray, the CT scan, and the bone scan are all designed to determine if the cancer has spread to your lymph nodes, bones, or other organs. The plates are fascinating to behold.

You have finally completed all the tests, and you have scheduled an appointment with your doctor to evaluate the results and decide on treatment. The "Preappointment Worksheet" on page 35 will help you assemble everything you should bring along to the appointment. (It may be preferable to have some results sent directly to your doctor.) Be sure to keep track of where everything is, since you will want to take all the records and reports with you. You will also want to assemble them again for your second opinion. (You will be reminded of this in the "Test Records II" worksheet on page 41.)

Before your appointment:

Step 1: Find out which records your first doctor will need. Place an "X" in the far-left column of the chart below, next to each required item.

Step 2: Indicate the current location of that record.

Step 3: If you want the record(s) sent to your doctor, find out if you can authorize release by phone.

Step 4: Determine when these records will be sent or when you can pick them up.

Step 5: If the office or lab will be sending the records, indicate the name of the person you talked with and how the records will be sent. If you pick them up, check the space in the "Picked up" column when you have them in your possession.

Step 6: If the records will be sent to your doctor, call a few days before your appointment to confirm that they were received. If you have them and are ready to take them with you, check the space in the "Received" column.

X	Records	Location	Phone release okay?	When?	Picked up or sent by	Received
☐	Medical history	Workbook	☐	_____	_____	☐
☐	Biopsy (histology) report	_____	☐	_____	_____	☐
☐	Ultrasound copies	_____	☐	_____	_____	☐
☐	Pathology reports	_____	☐	_____	_____	☐
☐	Pathology slides	_____	☐	_____	_____	☐
☐	X rays	_____	☐	_____	_____	☐
☐	Other	_____	☐	_____	_____	☐
☐	_____	_____	☐	_____	_____	☐
☐	_____	_____	☐	_____	_____	☐

Space for Your Notes:

....

....

....

....

PREAPPOINTMENT WORKSHEET

After you've undergone all the required tests, your doctor will make an appointment to discuss the results and your treatment alternatives. Check off in the list below those items you may need to take to the appointment.

☐ Workbook or applicable worksheets (see Chapter 6)

☐ Pencils, pen

☐ Tape recorder, cassette tape

☐ Location of appointment: _____

    Room #: _____ Time of appointment: _____

☐ Doctor's name: _____

☐ Name of doctor's staff member who made appointment: _____

☐ Doctor's phone number: _____

☐ Insurance cards

    Does doctor accept my insurance? ☐ Yes ☐ No

    If not, what payment is expected at the time of the visit? _____

☐ Credit cards

    Does the doctor accept credit cards? ☐ Yes ☐ No

    Which? _____

☐ General Medical History (see pages 25–29)

☐ List of questions

Space for Your Notes:

....

....

....

....

....

....

....

Space for Your Notes:

CHAPTER 6

Diagnosis and Treatment Protocols

"Now That I Have All the News, What Do I Do with It?"

All this testing and scanning is designed to tell your doctor exactly where the cancer is located and how virulent it is. You are now ready for your post-testing appointment, which is when you will get your first glimmer of what's in store for you. This appointment is an emotionally charged one. You will learn just how dangerous your cancer is. In addition, a course of treatment will be proposed here—one that will certainly change your life! I can't emphasize enough the importance of proper preparation for this meeting. Hopefully, you've done your homework and have all of the materials you will need.

It is vital that you have your partner at this meeting. A lot will be thrown at you, and you will need a second set of ears to catch it all. Again, I suggest you use the worksheet that follows and have your partner use the corresponding form in the back of the book.

Your doctor will review your status and the results of the tests. Your disease will be assigned a "stage" designation. For all the world, you hope for a good result. All of your future decisions will be based on the stage assigned.

At one time in the past, there were only four stages assigned to prostate cancer. There are now several subdivisions. At the risk of confusing a confusing topic even further, here is a simplified version of prostate cancer stages.

Stage A is what you hope for; this is when it has been determined that the tumors are very small and still wholly contained within the prostate gland. Before the advent of the PSA test, men lived for years with this stage of cancer undetected. Today, an elevated PSA alerts us that there is a problem, and a biopsy reveals this early stage.

Under the new system, stage A patients are assigned **stage T1** if no more than 5 percent of the biopsy sample is found to contain cancerous tissue. **Stage T2** means more than 5 percent is affected. The Gleason scale is also a factor in determining which stage is assigned.

Stage B tumors can be felt by the doctor with a digital rectal exam. These tumors are also confined to the prostate. Your doctor will use the test results and the size of the tumor to assign the new stage designation to your disease. The new designation is stage T2, which is further subdivided into T2/B1, B2, or B3:

- In **T2/B1,** the tumor is relatively small, but still palpable to the touch.

- **T2/B2** tumors are a bit larger, usually about half an inch wide, and confined to a small area of the prostate.

- **T2/B3** tumors have spread through both lobes of the prostate gland. Sometimes, if the tumors are small, a T2/B2 stage will be assigned even though both lobes are involved.

Stage C is the designation given when the cancer has spread out of the capsule of the prostate itself and into the adjacent tissues. In the new **stage T3,** the cancer has spread to tissue directly adjacent to the prostate or to the seminal vesicles. In **stage T4,** tumors have spread to organs a bit farther from the prostate, such as the bladder.

Stage D is denoted when the cancer has metastasized to other parts of the body. This means the prostate cancer cells have spread to the lymph nodes, bones, bladder, or lungs. It is important to note that in metastasizing, the cancer cells remain prostate cancer cells. They don't become liver cancer cells, for example. That is why additional PSA tests are given after treatment. This prostate-specific test will react positively if prostate cancer has spread undetected to other parts of the body.

The new system divides cancer that has spread into two categories. If it has spread to the lymph nodes in the pelvis, **stage D/N+** is denoted. If the cancer has spread to organs, bones, or lymph nodes farther from the prostate, **stage D/M+** is assigned. There are several subdivisions within these stage-D cancers:

- **D0** is used when the tests suggest that the cancer has progressed to either of the D stages, but there is no other evidence to indicate just where or how far.

- **D1** means that the cancer has spread to the nearby lymph nodes.

- **D2** indicates that the doctors have detected cancer not only in the lymph nodes, but in other parts of the body as delineated above (e.g., D/N+ or D/M+).

- The **D3** designation is used only after the patient has been treated for cancer, and the cancer has continued to spread.

Space for Your Notes:

After your various tests—such as bone scan, CT scan, and the like—the next appointment you'll have with your doctor is the most vital one you will face. The doctor will evaluate the test results and offer suggestions for treatment. Ask questions of the doctor, and write down (or tape-record, if he or she is comfortable with your doing so) all of the doctor's comments and answers. Your partner should do the same on the form provided on page 123 and compare notes with you later.

What is your assessment of my cancer? _____

What stage would you assign to it? _____

Is it self-contained? ☐ Yes ☐ No

How far has it spread? _____

What other parts of my body are affected? _____

What treatment options are open to me?

☐ Watchful waiting

☐ Hormone therapy

☐ Surgery

☐ Brachytherapy (seeds)

☐ External radiation

☐ Cryosurgery

☐ Other _____

Of the options open to me, what are the various risks? _____

_____

If you were I, which treatment would you choose? _____

_____

Before you leave this appointment, tell the doctor you think it prudent to obtain a second opinion and that you want to take all your records with you. (The "Test Records II" worksheet on page 41 will help you make sure you have all of the records you will need.)

First session notes:

....

....

....

....

Not all these may be needed, but it's easier to get them now.

Check before you leave your evaluation appointment that you have:

- ☐ Biopsy (histology) report
- ☐ Ultrasound copies
- ☐ Pathology reports
- ☐ Pathology slides
- ☐ X rays
- ☐ Other reports or test results

Space for Your Notes:

....

....

....

....

....

....

....

....

....

....

....

....

....

....

....

....

....

....

....

Your doctor has made his recommendations. You'll probably want to get a second opinion (see Chapter 7 for more information on this subject), but first, with your partner, if possible, review your options as outlined in your previous appointment. What now? Your comfort or discomfort, the length of your treatment—indeed, your life—will be affected by what you do in the next few months.

I strongly urge you to gather as much reliable information as you can. Your local bookstore or library will carry perhaps a dozen books on the subject of prostate cancer. The Internet is full of information, both reliable and off-the-wall. Remember that anyone can have an Internet site. Evaluate all information critically. I recommend some books and websites later in the book.

The best sources for me were other men who had faced this problem before. All of them, without exception, spent hours with me, sharing what they knew as a result of their experiences. If you can't find a buddy who's had prostate cancer, good support groups exist. To find one, check with your local hospital or contact some of the organizations listed on page 80 or in the Resources section beginning on page 136.

Several of the men I spoke with chose courses of treatment different from that which I opted for, and later on I'll discuss why they did so. The important thing at this stage is to gather as much information as you can to make an *informed* decision. Each man I spoke to who had followed this advice was happy with the outcome, irrespective of the treatment he'd selected.

If you are over age seventy or have serious medical problems, the prescribed course of action is **watchful waiting**. Prostate cancer *is* slow-moving, so, frankly, your chances of dying from a heart attack, or another cause, are greater than dying from cancer. The doctor I went to for a second opinion asked me about longevity in my family. I told him that my father was close to ninety. My grandparents also had lived into their eighties and nineties. I also told him that I had some truly exceptional grandchildren and that I wanted to increase my chances of living as long as I could. This doctor felt that, all things considered, my best chance of seeing them grow up meant undergoing a **radical prostatectomy** (the surgical solution).

One person on my advisory panel had opted for **external radiation therapy**. This is commonly the treatment of choice for men who prefer not to have surgery. He reported that the treatment was painless, but some of the aftereffects were unpleasant. Nausea is a common side effect, and because the radiation cannot be pinpointed precisely at the cancer cells, damage sometimes occurs to nearby healthy cells. A cousin of mine who had radiation therapy over ten years ago is still with us, with the help of additional hormone therapy.

Methods exist today for focusing external-radiation beams more precisely, but in my case the prostate was so large that there was a great risk of colon involvement. This did not rule out radiation treatment for me, but it was a big factor in my choosing another option.

Male hormones promote the growth of prostate cancer cells, so **hormone therapy**—the administration of estrogen—will most often arrest the growth of the cancer. Some patients opt for this course as their only therapy. Hormone therapy does not cure the cancer, and the treatment will probably be required for the rest of the patient's life. It is, however, an excellent choice for some patients, and it is a field in which research is progressing rapidly. It is also a viable option for patients whose cancer recurs at a later time as it can slow the progress of the disease.

I got a call one day from a friend of a friend. The caller spent an hour of long-distance time telling me of his experiences. He had opted for **brachytherapy,** the implantation of small radioactive pellets directly into the prostate. Each is about the size of a grain of rice and must be implanted very precisely. My caller had had to delay the implantation because of his business schedule, so he had undergone hormone therapy to slow the progress of the disease until the implantation could take place.

The success of brachytherapy is greatly dependent on the skill of the surgeon. It is used most often in early-stage cancers that are confined to a fairly specific area. Because the prostate must be relatively small, hormone therapy is sometimes used to shrink the size of the gland before brachytherapy. The surgeon is required to carefully space the implanted seeds for their greatest effect. He usually does this with sonographic aid. This is minor surgery and is done through the perineum (between the scrotum and anus).

Brachytherapy patients have the advantage of undergoing surgery on an outpatient basis. They are anesthetized, and then the seeds are implanted. There is no incision scar to deal with. The patient is usually released from the hospital the same day, usually as soon as he is able to urinate.

This treatment generally causes a loss of libido. Urination is sometimes painful, urgent, and frequent for a time after implantation. Brachytherapy patients report fewer bowel difficulties than do those who receive radiation. Fatigue is a common problem. Incontinence and impotence are also a possibility (these problems are dealt with in Chapter 14).

Brachytherapy patients worry about holding their grandchildren on their knee. There is no proven danger of exposing children to radioactivity in this way, and no such cases have been reported. It does seem wise, however, to limit the length of contact. Perhaps, for example, sitting a child on your lap to watch a long television show would be imprudent.

Chemotherapy is administered for advanced cases of cancer. This and other alternatives, such as **cryotherapy,** should be approached with knowledge. If you have questions about these alternatives, please consult some of the relevant resources listed at the back of this book (beginning on page 136).

Two or three viable treatments may exist for your stage of cancer. Making a decision may be hard, but the important thing is to weigh the pros and cons before you decide. That way, whatever you choose will be based on the facts. It will be the right choice for you to take control and mount war on your cancer.

For me, the two most viable treatments were external radiation therapy and a radical prostatectomy, that is, surgical removal of the entire gland. One of my buddies pointed out that if the surgery was unsuccessful, I could still opt for radiation. But if I opted for radiation and it was unsuccessful, there would probably be enough damage to the tissue around the prostate to preclude surgery. With my grandchildren in mind, and only after careful analysis of the pros and cons of each treatment, I decided to get rid of the monster. I chose to have a radical prostatectomy.

Take time now to note your reactions to what you know so far. Then, sit down with your partner and, using the "Treatment Option Evaluation" worksheets on pages 45 and 46, examine the pros and cons of each treatment offered to you.

List each option open to you, then write the positive factors of that option on one side of the chart; and the negative factors on the other side. Your doctor or the second-opinion physician should cover these issues. If he fails to do so, ask questions!

Option: _____

	Positive Factors	**Negative Factors**
Odds of cure:	_____	_____
	_____	_____
Length of treatment:	_____	_____
	_____	_____
Side effects:	_____	_____
	_____	_____
Risks:	_____	_____
	_____	_____
Other factors:	_____	_____

Option: _____

	Positive Factors	**Negative Factors**
Odds of cure:	_____	_____
	_____	_____
Length of treatment:	_____	_____
	_____	_____
Side effects:	_____	_____
	_____	_____
Risks:	_____	_____
	_____	_____
Other factors:	_____	_____

Option: _____

	Positive Factors	**Negative Factors**
Odds of cure:	_____	_____
	_____	_____
Length of treatment:	_____	_____
	_____	_____
Side effects:	_____	_____
	_____	_____
Risks:	_____	_____
	_____	_____
Other factors:	_____	_____

Option: _____

	Positive Factors	**Negative Factors**
Odds of cure:	_____	_____
	_____	_____
Length of treatment:	_____	_____
	_____	_____
Side effects:	_____	_____
	_____	_____
Risks:	_____	_____
	_____	_____
Other factors:	_____	_____

CHAPTER 7

Second Opinions

"Says Who?"

Because the prostate is connected to the urethra and because it is connected to the nerves that cause erection, the two most likely problems you will face after treatment are impotence and incontinence. In other words, you might not be able to have an erection, and you might have to wear pads or other urinary protection for the rest of your life.

If the idea of enduring either of these two problems doesn't bother you, put your hand out and let your doctor lead you where he will. If, on the other hand, you want to minimize the probabilities of these effects, you *must* make informed decisions at this time. Do not proceed from here blindly.

I wanted a second opinion. But first, I wanted to find the best cancer-treatment facility in my area. This was a daunting task, as many such facilities were located nearby. (The "Finding a Cancer-Treatment Facility" worksheet on page 49 will help you with this very important task.)

In most cases, the hospital's public-relations department sent me a packet of useful information about the facility. Most of the packets contained a map that showed the location of the cancer-treatment center, where to park, and so on. Several sent complete brochures outlining their philosophy of treatment, the number of cases of each type of cancer treated, and their success rate. A few hospitals actually had little experience treating cancer, having treated only a handful of prostate cancer cases. I eliminated those and came up with four hospitals that sounded good. I visited the post-op floors of each. One really looked ratty, and the nursing staff looked harried. That left me with three.

I started calling friends—and friends of friends—who had had recent hospital experience. One suggested that I choose one of our local hospitals. "They are heavily endowed," he said, "and the nurse-to-patient ratio is exceptional." Since I'd be seeing more of the nursing staff than the doctors, this made great sense. After further investigation and referrals, I did choose a local hospital. It turned out that the care was wonderful, and with my insurance it cost me no more than using one of the less-attractive or less-competent ones would have cost.

I asked for a list of urologists who practiced at this hospital. Several names coincided with referrals from my friends. I chose one and made an appointment for a second opinion. My regular urologist was an old-timer; he had given me fifty-fifty odds at best in the matters of impotence and incontinence. In addition to getting a second opinion, I wanted to know what I could do to increase those odds.

If your doctor offers resistance to your going for a second opinion, find another doctor! Ask your doctor if he wouldn't want a second opinion if he were in your shoes. Second opinions are not only your right, but they are highly recommended by the National Cancer Institute and are insisted on by many health-insurance organizations. (You will find the "Second-Opinion Questions" worksheet on page 50.)

If you have a choice of several therapies, you should also talk to physicians who practice each type. For example, talk to a radiologist if radiation therapy is a second option to a prostatectomy. Just keep in mind that each specialist will naturally favor the therapy he practices.

The second urologist I saw had several things in his favor. He carefully reviewed the tests, including my bone and CT scans. He gave me a lot of his time. He methodically reviewed all of the alternatives, including some I was hearing about for the first time.

In short, though he had performed many prostate operations, he was younger (under fifty) and more knowledgeable about the newer practices. He, like my first urologist, used the **Walsh method,** a protocol developed by Dr. Patrick Walsh of Johns Hopkins Medical School, that helps preserve the nerves involved with erections. This surgical procedure is sometimes called a "nerve-sparing operation." This second doctor had also developed a procedure that decreased the chances of permanent incontinence. The capper was when he did a digital exam on me. Though he seemed as thorough, I was far less uncomfortable than with my previous doctor. His recommendation was the same as the first doctor's—radical prostatectomy.

Adding up all the pieces—his age, his manner, the number of prostatectomy operations he had performed, and the hospital where he practiced—I decided to bite the bullet and have him do the deed as quickly as possible.

FINDING A CANCER-TREATMENT FACILITY

How close is the facility to my home? _____

How many prostate cancer cases does it treat each year? _____

How many prostatectomies does it perform? _____

How many are treated with radiation? _____

What has been its mortality rate? _____

How does that compare with the national average? _____

Does the facility have the ability to do all my testing on-site, including:

☐ Blood work?

☐ CT scans?

☐ Bone scans?

☐ X rays?

What other services does the facility provide?

☐ Nutritionist?

☐ Cancer support group?

☐ Psychological help?

☐ Chaplaincy services?

☐ Social workers?

Other services available: _____

_____

What is the nurse-to-patient ratio? _____

Is care at this facility covered by my health insurance? ☐ Yes ☐ No

What portions and how much of my bill will be covered? _____

_____

What arrangements are available for the payment of the balance? _____

_____

Space for Your Notes:

....

....

....

SECOND-OPINION QUESTIONS

For discussion with a second-opinion doctor:

After reviewing my records, what is your assessment of my cancer? _____

_____

_____

What treatment options are open to me?

- ☐ Watchful waiting

- ☐ Hormone therapy

- ☐ Surgery

- ☐ Brachytherapy (seeds)

- ☐ External radiation

- ☐ Cryosurgery

Other options: _____

Of the open options, what are my odds? _____

_____

Of the open options, what are my risks? _____

_____

If you were I, which treatment would you choose? _____

_____

_____

Space for Your Notes:

....

....

....

....

....

....

....

....

(Second Opinion)

Again, list each option open to you; then write the positive factors of that option on one side of the chart and the negative factors on the other side. Your doctor or the second-opinion physician should cover these issues. If he fails to do so, ask questions!

Option: _____

	Positive Factors	**Negative Factors**
Odds of cure:	_____	_____
	_____	_____
Length of treatment:	_____	_____
	_____	_____
Side effects:	_____	_____
	_____	_____
Risks:	_____	_____
	_____	_____
Other factors:	_____	_____

Option: _____

	Positive Factors	**Negative Factors**
Odds of cure:	_____	_____
	_____	_____
Length of treatment:	_____	_____
	_____	_____
Side effects:	_____	_____
	_____	_____
Risks:	_____	_____
	_____	_____
Other factors:	_____	_____

Option: _____

	Positive Factors	**Negative Factors**
Odds of cure:	_____	_____
	_____	_____
Length of treatment:	_____	_____
	_____	_____
Side effects:	_____	_____
	_____	_____
Risks:	_____	_____
	_____	_____
Other factors:	_____	_____

Option: _____

	Positive Factors	**Negative Factors**
Odds of cure:	_____	_____
	_____	_____
Length of treatment:	_____	_____
	_____	_____
Side effects:	_____	_____
	_____	_____
Risks:	_____	_____
	_____	_____
Other factors:	_____	_____

During this appointment with your second-opinion doctor, you may want to review the assessments you made after your first post-testing doctor's appointment (see the first "Treatment Option Evaluation" worksheet on pages 45–46). Does the new doctor agree with your assessment?

CHAPTER 8

Supplementary Therapies

"Quack, Quack?"

While I was investigating all my options, lots of ideas were tossed on the table. One friend took my cancer as a personal insult and mounted a campaign against it. He wanted me to try anything that would increase my chances. This included yoga and a macrobiotic diet. Others suggested, in rapid succession, the herbal supplements St. John's wort, echinacea, and saw palmetto, some of which, I learned from my research, could have turned out to be counterproductive! Saw palmetto, for example, can lower PSA results, thereby masking a possibly serious problem. I took none of these supplements, but I did feel there were certain steps I could take on my own—that is, outside the scope of my official, doctor-supervised medical care— that would help in my treatment and general well-being.

I felt that anything I could do to improve my immune system would be helpful. I had some bad habits. I was a six-pack-a-day Diet Coke drinker. I certainly didn't need that artificial sweetener in my system, so I cut it out. (My Coke stock subsequently took a big dip. I blamed it on my disease.) I was fat and flabby, so I started to walk daily in an effort to increase my stamina. If I'd had more time, I would have joined a gym and worked out. I also asked for suggestions from dieticians.

I checked and cross-checked all recommendations with my doctors. They often pooh-poohed a course of action, but I always asked, "Will it hurt me?" If they said no, I considered it further, knowing that, by training, physicians must be conservative. Some of the things I asked about, such as the use of saw palmetto and the benefits of eating bean sprouts, were judged by the doctor to be definitely harmful, and I crossed them off the list. (Sprouts are thought to be carriers of bacteria.)

My very cautious internist felt that some of the suggested techniques and cures, including wearing copper bracelets, were quackery, but I always asked him, "How will it hurt me?" If he deemed it harmful, I discarded the idea, but if his answer was vague, I investigated the efficacy of the idea further. I felt that I should rely on modern medicine for my treatment, but that certain other therapies might *complement* the traditional treatment. Perhaps they would even help significantly.

As it turned out, two complementary therapies proved most helpful in my case. Relaxation exercises made me more comfortable in some rather tense situations and got me through the few times when I needed pain management. Walking, both before and after the operation, speeded my recovery, and while it didn't help my physique much, it did make me stronger when I needed to be.

Other disciplines exist that you might like to investigate. A list follows, with suggestions about where to go for further information.

Acupressure

Think of acupressure as acupuncture without the needles.

To locate a practitioner, contact the American Oriental Bodywork Therapy Association in Voorhees, NJ; website: www.healthy.net/pan/pa/bodywork/

Books:

Kenyon, Julian, *Acupressure Techniques: A Self-Help Guide.* Rochester, VT: Inner Traditions International, 1996.

Young, Jacqueline, *Acupressure Step by Step: The Oriental Way to Health.* London: Thorsons, 1998.

Acupuncture

A traditional Chinese system of medicine, this relatively painless practice can produce a deep sense of relaxation and relief from chronic pain.

Your local yellow pages might contain a list of practitioners. Or call the American Association of Oriental Medicine in Catasauqua, Pennsylvania; tel. (610) 433-2448. The Acupuncture and Oriental Medicine Alliance in Olalla, Washington, maintains a website: www.acuall.org.

Books:

Fleischman, Gary F., and Charles Stein, *Acupuncture: Everything You Ever Wanted to Know but Were Afraid to Ask*. Barrytown, NY: Barrytown, Ltd., 1998.

Journaling

Consider keeping a notebook recording your plans, feelings, and thoughts. Journaling works best if done in an organized, disciplined fashion for half an hour or so each day.

Books:

Bender, Sheila, *A Year in the Life: Journaling for Self-Discovery*. Cincinnati, OH: Writer's Digest Books, 2000.

Ganim, Barbara, and Susan Fox, *Visual Journaling: Going Deeper than Words*. Wheaton, IL: Quest Books, 1999.

Massage and Body Therapy

There are over a hundred different types of massage, ranging from Alexander technique to rolfing. You instinctively massage yourself when you knead a sore muscle.

Certified massage therapists are listed in the yellow pages; they also advertise in magazines available at most health-food stores. As an additional resource, the American Massage Therapy Association in Evanston, Illinois, can be reached at (847) 864-0123 or on its website at www.amtamassage.org.

Books:

Capellini, Steve, and Michael van Welden, *Massage for Dummies*. New York: Hungry Minds, 1999.

Lidell, Lucinda, *The Book of Massage*. New York: Fireside, 2001.

Meditation

Meditation offers a way to focus the mind on the quiet present.

The Harvard Medical School offers classes, information, and referral in transcendental meditation at the Mind/Body Clinic of the New Deaconess Hospital. Contact The Mind/Body Medical Clinic at

Beth Israel Deaconess Medical Center, 110 Francis St., Ste. 1A, Boston, MA 02215. (617) 632-9530, press 1. For an Internet resource, see its website at www.mbmi.org/pages/mp_csas1.asp.

Books:

Bodian, Stephan, *Meditation for Dummies*. New York: Hungry Minds, 1999.

Harris, Rachel, *20-Minute Retreats: Revive Your Spirit in Just Minutes a Day with Simple Self-Led Practices*. New York: Owl Books, 2000.

Quigong

(pronounced—and sometimes spelled—"chi-kung")

Tai chi is a well-known, slow-moving martial art branch of quigong that has its roots in Taoist meditation. Quigong involves deliberate, dancelike movements that engender a state of meditation and relaxation.

Quigong is taught at community centers, hospitals, and colleges. Check with your local YMCA, or visit the website of the East–West Academy of Oriental Arts: www.eastwestqi.com.

Books:

Chu, Vincent, *Beginner's Tai Chi Chuan*. Burbank, CA: Multi-Media Books, 2000.

David, Catherine, and Alison Anderson (translator), *The Beauty of Gesture: The Invisible Keyboard of Piano and T'ai Chi*. Berkeley, CA: North Atlantic Books, 1996.

Jahnke, Roger, *The Healer Within*. San Francisco, CA: Harper San Francixco, 1999.

Relaxation

This practice teaches your body to relax on cue.

Books:

Benson, Herbert, *The Relaxation Response*. New York: Avon Books, 1990.

Benson, Herbert, and William Procter, *Beyond the Relaxation Response*. New York: Berkley Books, 1994.

Davis, Martha, Matthew McKay, and Elizabeth Robbins Eshelman, *The Relaxation and Stress-Reduction Workbook.* Oakland, CA: New Harbinger, 2000.

Lazarus, Judith, *Stress Relief and Relaxation Techniques.* New York: McGraw-Hill, 2000.

Tai Chi

See *quigong*.

Walking

The easiest form of exercise, walking is also among the most beneficial.

Books and tapes:

Fenton, Mark, and Seth Bauer, *The 90-Day Fitness Walking Program.* New York: Perigree, 1995.

Moreno, Rita, and the American Heart Association, *The Healthy Heart Walking Tape: Walking Workouts for a Lifetime of Fitness* (audiocassette). New York: Simon & Schuster (Audio), 1996.

Neporent, Liz, *Fitness Walking for Dummies.* New York: Hungry Minds, 1999.

Yoga

Yoga is a widely taught discipline of stretching exercises that merge mind, body, and spirit. To locate classes, check your local adult education programs, as well as magazines at most health food stores.

The website www.yogamusicvideo.com offers yoga books, videos, etc.

Books:

Feuerstein, Georg, Larry Payne, and Lilias Folan, *Yoga for Dummies.* New York: Hungry Minds, 1999.

Space for Your Notes:

CHAPTER 9

Family, Sex, and the Law

"What Do I Tell My Grandkids?"

I have some exceptional grandchildren (don't we all?). They range in age from one to thirteen, and they are all beautiful, smart, and sensitive. I wanted them and their parents to be prepared for what was going to happen. Each spring we celebrate Passover, and I write my own service. At the Seder, which took place a few weeks before my operation, I spoke to my family about my illness. You might choose Easter dinner or just call the family together or write a letter or do it individually, but don't hide your disease. Prostate cancer is not the shame it was when you were a kid. You owe it to your loved ones to be open, optimistic, and realistic.

To plan what to say to my family, I generally followed the outline suggested by Barbara Rubin Wainrib and Sandra Haber in their helpful book, *Men, Women, and Prostate Cancer*. Here is what I said:

> *The doctors tell me that I'm seriously sick, but they're very confident that they can make me well. You can't catch this disease. It's not spread by sneezing or by a bug. Sometimes it makes me extremely tired, but other than that, I feel just fine. If I don't take care of it, however, I will get very sick.*
>
> *I am in the process of getting tests done, donating blood for myself, and learning everything I can about my illness. On May eighth, I will go to Bryn Mawr Hospital for three or four days. While I'm there, a great guy, Dr. Squadrito, will operate on me and remove the disease from my body.*

There will be times after the operation when I will not be feeling very well, and I may be sad or grouchy. I want you to be very patient with me. Please come and keep me company after the operation, but if I ask you to leave, please know that it is nothing you've done; I'm just feeling tired or in pain. Grandmom Rina is my Chief of Support, and she will take good care of me.

I have lots of other people who are on my support team. I regularly get calls from Murray and Debby offering very helpful suggestions. Essie called with her usual good sense, humor, and great advice. We found Dr. Squadrito through her. Myrna and Richard have been key members of the support team. Walter Ferst, our constant friend, has had a lot of experience with this sickness. He has helped in many ways, not the least of which are his good common-sense doses of reality.

I get e-mail from the Solars, Ruth Brott, Marty and Phyllis Cohen, and many more. I consult with Dick Gross, who had the same operation eight weeks ago. He has been most generous with his advice and time. Ruth and Rudy Lea call to check on us, and Len and Elaine Cohen have regularly called in with suggestions and caring advice. All of this is very important to me.

If you consider the names I've just mentioned and look around this table, you will see that I have a lot of help in dealing with this illness.

Jordan and Callan and Julian have brought such joy to me. Rob, Jamie, Amanda, and Adam have been very supportive. Each of you is so unique and wonderful. I look forward with optimism and joy to watching you all blossom and do great things with your lives.

I don't want you to worry about me. There are plenty of folks who are doing that and who are helping me get the best care I can possibly get. You know how much I love you and your smiling faces. Those smiles will be the best way for you to help me get better fast.

Things Your Family Might Worry About

Try to reassure your family in your letter or your talk with them. They will probably want to know the following:

- Are you in pain?

- Will you die?

- Is it contagious? Will I get it?

- What do the doctors say?

- How are you going to get better?

- Where?

- When?

- Who is the doctor?

- How will you feel after your treatment?

- How long will it take?

- Who is in charge? Name names.

- What other help are you getting?

- Who else knows about this, and how do they feel about it?

- Can we visit you? Do we have to wait until you come home from the hospital?

- How will you feel when we do?

- What do you expect from us?

- What do you want me to say?

- What do you want me NOT to say?

- What do you want me to ask?

- What do you want me NOT to ask?

- How can we help?

Make notes here about your family's specific worries:

....

....

....

BLOOD ISSUES

My surgery was three weeks away. I had a lot to think about and do. One of these concerns was the safety of the blood used during my surgery. Since the advent of AIDS, this has become a real issue. While extraordinary measures are taken to ensure that the blood supply is safe, you are safest if the hospital has a supply of your own blood. I needed to contribute three units of blood to myself in case it would be needed during the operation.

I started taking iron supplements immediately. The maximum you can donate is one unit per week, so we were playing it a bit close. I reported to the Red Cross on the appointed day, filled out all the forms, had my temperature taken, and my finger pricked to draw a drop of blood to test for iron content. I also signed the necessary papers to ensure that my own blood would show up at the correct hospital on the day of my surgery. I lay on the couch, and a tourniquet was placed on my upper arm. The nurse swabbed iodine on the inner arm where the needle was to go. Uh oh! Little pimples erupted.

They tried the other arm. Same problem. They refused to take my blood, saying the pimples might indicate an infection. The last thing I needed was to transfuse an infection into my system after an operation. They could not schedule another appointment before the one I'd already made for a week later. That left me short one unit.

I called the urologist, who assured me this was not a major problem. He suggested I tell the technicians drawing blood not to use latex gloves and not to use iodine to disinfect the contribution site because I might be allergic to both.

The second attempt went like clockwork. Whew! They tagged my blood, gave me the corresponding number to take to the hospital, fed me a drink of juice, and I went gratefully on my way.

The day I was scheduled to give my third unit turned out to be very hot. On my way to the Red Cross, the air conditioner in my car died. I arrived there rather hot and bothered. I went through the same predonation routine. This time I was running a slightly elevated temperature. I sat out another half hour, and my temperature dropped a fraction, but it was still above the Red Cross guidelines. I was unable to convince them that they should take my blood anyway.

I was in the position of going into a major operation with only one unit of my own blood. If I needed more, I would have to get it from the donated pool. The doctor said I would probably not need it and reemphasized that stringent tests and controls are in place to control the quality and safety of donated blood. I could have deferred the operation, but the next available date was over six months away. I didn't want to risk the possibility of the cancer spreading.

In fact, I did lose a lot of blood during the operation. However, aside from feeling beat up from the surgery and being a bit anemic, I did not feel too bad from the loss of blood. Nonetheless, since my one unit of blood was available, I was transfused with it the day after my operation. This procedure can take hours, but since you are still hooked up to an IV, you won't have to have another needle stuck into you. They simply plug the tube into the hardware that's already there. I was anemic for a month or so after the operation, but aside from being tired from time to time, the one unit, plus some supplementary iron pills, proved sufficient.

My advice is that you start the self-donation process as soon as you know that you are going ahead with surgery. Another option, especially if you have an unusual blood type, is to line up friends who could be prospective donors if needed. You never know what difficulties you may encounter, so give yourself as much time to do these things as you can.

BLOOD-DONATION APPOINTMENTS

X	Date	Location	Done
☐	_____	_____	_____
☐	_____	_____	_____
☐	_____	_____	_____
☐	_____	_____	_____
☐	_____	_____	_____
☐	_____	_____	_____

POST–BLOOD DONATION CHECKLIST

☐ Drink four extra glasses of nonalcoholic liquids (eight ounces each).

☐ Keep bandage on and dry for five hours after donation.

☐ No heavy exercise or heavy lifting for rest of day.

☐ If dizzy, lie down and raise your feet.

☐ If needle site starts to bleed, raise your arm straight up and press the needle-insertion area until the bleeding stops.

☐ Follow safety recommendations before returning to work. You could experience dizziness or weakness.

☐ You might have a multicolored bruise for up to ten days after donation. If you get a bruise, apply ice for ten to fifteen minutes every half hour or so for the first day. After that, intermittently apply warm, moist heat to the area for ten to fifteen minutes.

Call the blood-donor center if:

☐ You get a bruise larger than two or three inches in diameter

☐ You have redness, swelling, or pain at the needle-insertion area

☐ You experience tingling in your fingers or arm

☐ You can't make the next appointment

Space for Your Notes:

....

....

....

YOUR TEETH, YOUR DIET, AND OTHER ISSUES
OF GENERAL HEALTH

Addressing certain other issues, such as dental and dietary concerns, will turn the odds in your favor for a speedy recovery. This is especially true if you are undergoing radiation therapy. Your immune system will be depressed, and you don't want an infected tooth to do you in. If you are having surgery, you don't want to have to deal with a toothache as well as your convalescence.

For these reasons, make a dental appointment as early as possible before your treatment begins. Inform your dentist about the mode of treatment you will be undergoing and when the treatment will occur. Your dentist should clean your teeth and repair anything that may be a problem later.

Many old-time doctors completely ignore the role of diet in cancer treatment. If this describes your doctor, it will remain up to you to make sure you're eating in a way that will strengthen rather than undermine your immune system. Some hospitals routinely schedule an appointment with a staff dietician. If not, make an appointment on your own with a good nutritionist. Doing so will help you untangle the confusing and sometimes conflicting advice about food and diet so widely available these days; you may also learn some new habits that you choose to embrace for long-term benefits in your changing lifestyle. Improving your diet is a matter for which you and your caregivers should take responsibility. At the very least, it will aid in your general well-being. It certainly won't hurt.

Eat a lot of high-fiber, low-fat foods. Dairy products, eggs, red meat, and saturated vegetable oils should be eaten sparingly or not at all. Instead, use unsaturated oils like olive or peanut oil, and eat plenty of cereals and whole-grain products. Michael Milken believes that a soy diet helped cure him of cancer. He maintains an extensive and informative website called CaP Cure (www.capcure.org).

If you smoke, this is a good time to quit. Scare yourself a little, and visualize yourself in a coffin whenever you pick up a cigarette. Some therapies will require you to cut out cigarettes and alcohol entirely.

As mentioned earlier, I was a six-pack-a-day Diet Coke drinker. When I was diagnosed with cancer, I stopped drinking it. I also stopped using artificial sweeteners and everything else I could that contained chemical additives. You really don't need all that caffeine and all those chemicals in your system while your body is fighting cancer.

It just makes good sense at this time that you want to rid your body of anything foreign. Try to return your body to as natural a state as you can by eating foods in forms close to how they came out of the earth (for example, choose whole-grain breads over the more processed white-flour bread, or fresh fruits over the canned variety). At the same time, approach "health" foods with investigative skepticism. Some foods that are favored by health-food stores, like sprouts of all kinds, are highly suspect as carriers of bacteria. You certainly don't want that in your system in the weeks ahead.

Ask your doctor about the role of antioxidants. These are substances that aid healthy cell growth and buttress the immune system. They are found naturally in leafy green vegetables such as spinach and Brussels sprouts, in fresh fruits, and in whole grains.

If you are a radiation patient, several other suggestions may make good sense. Let your doctor know if you are feeling nauseated or even mildly queasy. He or she can give you medicine that will help. Cut out gas-producing foods. Eat a number of small meals instead of the traditional three a day. Eat when you feel the need to, not by the clock. You might want to carry snacks with you when you go out.

In any event, if you face problems related to your diet, consult with your doctor or dietician. There is much you can do to help yourself.

For general well-being, especially for radiation and surgery patients, a good exercise program also makes sense. If nothing else, get in the habit of taking long walks.

LEGAL ISSUES

A cancer diagnosis does not mean that you will die from the disease, but you do want to be sure you have all your ducks in a row. My estate was not complicated, and no changes to my will were necessary. I did, however, have some definite feelings about quality-of-life issues. I wanted to leave clear instructions for my family and my doctors in the event of my death or permanent disability.

If the operation did not go well, if I became terminally ill or disabled, or if I became a vegetable, I did not want measures taken to keep me alive. I have lived through situations where families were subjected to months and years of anguish, and to financial hardship, all in the name of a hopeless cause. My own father had lived for more than two years with great pain before he died. My mother valiantly nursed him at home at great peril to her own health.

I did not fear death. I have lived a good life with a wonderful wife and a loving family. I have been especially blessed with the love of my grandchildren. I *did* want to live as long as possible so that I could see them grow up. I did not, however, want their last remembrance of me to be an unhappy one.

If my health became irreparable, I wanted to die as quickly as possible. The legal instrument for ensuring that this will happen is called an **advance directive**—sometimes called a **living will,** a **durable health-care power of attorney,** or a **health-care proxy.** The terms are interchangeable, but each state has its preferred designation. All facilities receiving medical funds from the federal government are required to tell you of your right to make such a determination. When this issue was brought up during my pre-op testing, I produced a signed and executed copy and asked that it be attached to my records.

When I told my internist that I was contemplating a living will, he counseled against it. It went counter to his training and nature. He told me several stories where living wills failed to do the patient any good. In one, a woman's two sons could not agree when her case was hopeless. One son, a lawyer, wanted the mother put out of her misery. The other son, a doctor, wanted every possible measure employed to keep his mother alive.

I listened carefully, and on the basis of his advice, I did temper the conditions of my living will. He had opined that it was a terrible thing for a family to decide to withhold life support from a loved one. I agreed. As a result, I chose as trustee of the will a levelheaded friend who I knew loved me and my family. I felt that he would be in a better position to make such a decision. I also discussed this decision with my family. Of course, I first asked my designated trustee if he would perform such a service for me. I gave him a copy of the will and went over every clause to make sure there was no question as to my intent.

A living will is not a complicated document, but each state has its own provisions for its makeup. Sources are available to help you. You can do your own, or your lawyer can draw one up for you in a jiffy.

Some suggested provisions for a living will are provided in the "Living-Will Worksheet" on pages 68–69.

Check with your hospital as to their policies concerning such directives. If they refuse to honor your wishes in this regard, you should find another hospital!

These provisions appeared in my living will, which was generated by the computer program *Family Lawyer*. Use them as a checklist to make sure your living will reflects your wishes precisely.

☐ I direct my attending physicians to withhold or withdraw life-sustaining treatment that serves only to prolong the process of my dying, if I should be in a terminal condition.

☐ I also direct my attending physicians to withhold or withdraw life-sustaining treatment that serves only to prolong the process of my dying, if I should be in a state of permanent unconsciousness.

☐ I direct that treatment be limited to measures to keep me comfortable and to relieve pain, including any pain that might occur by withholding or withdrawing life-sustaining treatment.

☐ If I have a condition stated above, it is my preference not to receive tube feeding or any other artificial or invasive form of nutrition or hydration (food or water).

☐ In addition, if I have a condition stated above, I direct that the following forms of treatment be avoided:

☐ I do not want cardiac resuscitation.

☐ I do not want blood or blood products.

☐ I do not want mechanical respiration.

☐ I do not want antibiotics or other therapeutic medicines.

☐ I do not want dialysis.

☐ I do not want any surgery.

☐ I do not want any invasive procedures or tests.

☐ If I should be incompetent and in a condition stated above, I designate

_____,

currently residing at_____,

as my surrogate to make medical-treatment decisions for me. If he/she is unable to serve,

I designate _____,

currently residing at_____,

as my surrogate.

© 2001 Broderbund Properties LLC

I have discussed my living-will issues with the following people:

Person   **Date**

Trustees: _____   _____

_____   _____

Lawyer: _____   _____

Doctors: _____   _____

_____   _____

_____   _____

_____   _____

Hospital: _____   _____

_____   _____

_____   _____

Family: _____   _____

_____   _____

_____   _____

_____   _____

_____   _____

_____   _____

Friends: _____   _____

_____   _____

_____   _____

_____   _____

_____   _____

_____   _____

_____   _____

_____   _____

_____   _____

SEX ISSUES

A close friend called to see if he could be of any help. I knew that he had undergone treatment for cancer of a different type. I asked for any words of wisdom. "Do you know about the birds and the bees?" he asked. "Of course," I answered. "Why?" He then gave me a piece of advice that I pass on to you.

He said that when he thought he might die, it lent a depth of meaning to the act of love. His episodes of lovemaking before his operation were rich and invested with deep meaning for him. After his operation, he lost interest in sex for a long period. His wife was most understanding, and he was able to express his love in other ways, but he was happy that he had enjoyed new depths of experience before the operation.

Do a lot of cuddling with your partner. That kind of intimacy will be more important later when it may be the only physical contact you are able to share. Impotence is not inevitable with this disease, but it is something to be considered. If you do become impotent, there is much you can do. These alternatives are discussed on pages 102–104.

Meanwhile, during these pretreatment days, my advice to you is this: Woo your wife or partner while you can. Squeeze as much physical love into your life as is possible. It will be a while before you are able to enjoy normal sexual relations with your partner. Store it up now.

Also, if you are in a position where you may want to have children in the future, talk to your doctor about banking some of your sperm—just in case.

CHAPTER 10

Operation Preparations

"You Want to Know *What?*"

Sometime before your operation, you will visit the hospital on an outpatient basis for your preoperation exam. You will be asked a hundred questions. Be ready! For your own health and safety, prepare for this examination as you did for your final exams when you were in school. If you haven't yet completed the "General Medical History" worksheet on pages 25–29, do so now. If you have already completed it, review it carefully.

Even if you don't use the forms provided in this book, write down your medical history. If you don't remember when you had your tonsils out, or if you can't find someone who might know, be prepared with an educated guess. If your parents had any major medical problems, you will want a list of what and when. In the rush of answering questions about my medical history, I remembered to tell them about my vascular surgery but forgot all about my vasectomy. Having a thorough medical history before me that I had prepared ahead of time, in the relaxed setting of my own home, would have been helpful. That's why I've included one in this book.

It is important to list anything to which you are allergic. This includes foods, medicines (e.g., penicillin, iodine), dust, dander, etc.

Most important, make a list of any pills you take. This includes aspirin and vitamins. If you take a multivitamin, copy the *contents* of that pill onto your list. If you take herbal supplements, make sure to list them. Better yet, consider carrying with you to the pre-op exam the bottles of all the pills you take. That way, the nurses and doctors can review the labels themselves. Some common herbs and multivitamin contents can get you into trouble.

Bring your list of questions. Most will be answered in the course of your day, but make sure you don't leave without getting all the answers you need. You will also, of course, need your health-insurance papers and a copy of your living will. You may be asked not to eat breakfast before the pre-op exam.

When you first arrive, an admissions officer will sign you in and take some administrative information. If they don't ask you about a living will, tell them you have one and would like to make it a part of your records. Give them a copy. Another copy should go to your doctor.

Next, you will undergo a series of tests and consultations. Included may be any or all of the procedures listed below.

Someone will take blood for your **blood tests**. A tight tourniquet will be placed around your upper arm, and a needle will be inserted at the inner elbow. If your veins are small or tend to collapse, ask the technician to use a pediatric needle. Despite the fact that a whole battery of tests will be done on your blood, you will only be stuck once.

You will have a meeting with an **anesthesiologist,** who will want to discuss any previous operations you have had with you. He or she will tell you the anesthesiology procedure particular to this hospital. (The usual drill is reviewed on pages 82–83.)

A nurse will take a thorough **medical history**. You will be asked many questions, and because you've carefully prepared as outlined above, you will ace this exam. If you are not asked a question you've prepared for (for example, whether you are taking herbal supplements), be sure that the nurse is informed of every last detail. You'll whip out your lists and he or she will look at you with great admiration. Most important, you will be protected from unexpected side effects, conditions, or drug interactions.

After your medical history is taken, **procedural matters** regarding your upcoming surgery and hospital stay will be reviewed. You'll be told to wear comfortable clothing and to leave your valuables at home. Visitation policies will be discussed. I asked if my grandkids could visit. The nurse said that the older ones could, but that I would not want them there the first day and would probably not be in the mood to see them until I got home. The nurse will probably also review with you all of the gadgets that will be a part of your post-op life in the hospital (discussed on pages 83–84).

You will likely get a standard **chest X ray.**

Each time you see someone new during your pre-op hospital visit, double-check your list to make sure your questions are answered. Consider giving each health-care professional you deal with that day a copy of your list beforehand. They are busy folks, and they will appreciate the fact that you have come prepared. It makes for a thorough and expedited procedure.

In my case, the hospital had its preoperation procedure planned down to the tiniest detail. They covered everything. When the technician who took my blood for testing left my side, a minute did not pass before the next professional entered the room. It was an amazing and welcome performance. I had virtually no time to read the book I had brought, and I was out within an hour and a half.

PREOPERATIVE EXAM CHECKLIST

Take with you:

- ☐ Insurance cards
- ☐ General Medical History (review it first)
- ☐ Copy of living will, advance directive, or health-care proxy
- ☐ List of questions
- ☐ List of dietary restrictions

Questions you might want to ask:

Where and when do I report?_____

What should I wear? _____

Anything else I should bring or leave at home? _____

How long will I be here? _____

Does my insurance cover everything? ☐ Yes ☐ No

If not, what is my responsibility? _____

Can I make special payment arrangements? ☐ Yes ☐ No

How will my partner be advised of my condition? _____

After the operation, when can I see my partner?_____

When can family members visit? _____

Can my grandchildren visit? ☐ Yes ☐ No When? _____

Other questions:

....

....

....

....

....

....

....

....

....

....

PERSONAL PREOPERATION PREPARATIONS

There are other things you can do to prepare for surgery. Your doctors probably won't discuss these with you, but I highly recommend that you review the suggestions below.

The first is to build up your strength. You want to be in the best physical condition possible for your operation. I increased the lengths of my habitual walks. I contemplated joining a gym, rejected the idea, and was later sorry I did. As your operation date nears, avoid people with colds and contagious diseases. This is just good common sense.

Understand that you will find yourself in some strange and tension-filled situations during the months ahead. Now is the time to prepare for them. I knew, for example, that many medications make me groggy. Even antihistamines make my head fuzzy for a full day after I take them. I'd learned from my buddies' panel that the pain reliever of choice following prostate surgery contained codeine. Codeine not only is habit-forming, but was sure to give me a hangover. I wanted some alternative way to control my pain. A psychologist friend recommended that I go to a hypnotist who specialized in pain conditioning. I found three in our local yellow pages.

The job of the hypnotist is to teach you *self*-hypnosis. You want to be able to visualize a stress-free environment that helps you take yourself away from the pain. Learning these skills takes time. I had very little of it before my scheduled surgery, so I regrettably had to forgo the hypnotism lessons.

In the past, however, I had taken relaxation training. The method of deep relaxation perfected at Harvard Medical Center and Beth Israel Hospital in Boston aims at helping a person enter the relaxation response by a conditioned reflex. For me, that reflex was triggered by tensing my wrist and fist as tightly as I could and then releasing it. When I released, my entire body relaxed. This technique also takes instruction and time, and I had not practiced in a few years.

My friend suggested that I systematically practice my relaxation techniques before the procedure. She also suggested other techniques to handle any pain or discomfort I might experience. I spent the next few weeks practicing and was very happy I did.

I am not very brave when it comes to this kind of experience. When I was prepped and waiting to go into the operating room, I experienced a panic attack. I quickly flexed my wrist, and the relaxation response kicked in, allowing me to calmly relax. These techniques also paid off in the area of pain management. After leaving the hospital, I was easily able to manage my pain with only Tylenol.

Other disciplines exist that can help with pain control and stress management. A few of my friends who'd experienced surgery practiced meditation. They reported that it was a great help. Whatever you choose, I suggest that you use at least one of these techniques. For other suggestions, refer to the list of supplementary therapies on pages 54–57. Please remember, though, that these techniques must be thought of as *supplements* to your treatment, not alternatives. Approach alternatives with skepticism. They can be most helpful, and even life-enhancing, but they will not cure your cancer.

Pick one or two of these disciplines for use even after your treatment. They can be helpful in regaining perspective and recentering yourself. You'll find use for them throughout the remainder of your life.

DEPRESSION

At some point in this process, you are going to feel very vulnerable. Suddenly, you face your own mortality. For some people, the blues hit almost immediately. Others experience deep depression during and after their treatment.

Sadness is a common response in general to major life upsets, and cancer is certainly something one might get depressed about. A significant percentage of cancer patients report being depressed at some point in their illness.

I was handling my diagnosis pretty well, when suddenly it hit me that I was really the person who was under attack by this disease. I got up from my desk in great agitation, started pacing the floor, then put my back against the wall and began to weep. I wept for the injustice of the attack. I wept for what I hadn't yet done with my life. I wept for all the things I'd left unsaid to friends and family and for all the places in the world I had not seen. I wept because I was just plain blue. I realized I had a right to be downhearted, but I didn't want the sadness to plunge me into depression. I didn't want to feel helpless and hopeless.

For the first time in decades, I wept deeply and long. Then, finally, I was able to focus on all the good things in my life: my wonderful marriage, my children, all my accomplishments, and all my friends. I was able to concentrate on the task at hand—on everything I needed to do to fight this thing.

This is not to say that I avoided experiencing mood swings. After surgery, and especially when dealing with impotence and incontinence, I often felt blue. From time to time I felt angry, sad, out of control, fearful, depressed, and eerie ("This can't be happening to me!"). From time to time I felt that certain mundane tasks, like paying bills, were impossible to accomplish. There were times when I couldn't put two thoughts together. I slept fitfully, felt too tired to do anything real, and immersed myself in computer games.

It is important that you recognize that all these responses are common among cancer patients and that you can do something about them when and if they occur. After all, you are now dealing with a lot of uncertainty and stress, not to mention some real fear.

First and foremost, discuss your feelings with your doctor and nurses. They will offer helpful suggestions, and perhaps medication if it is indicated. In addition to seeking advice, it is helpful to take proactive command of your disease and its treatment. By the time you have reached this chapter, you are well on your way to doing this.

There are many great resources for dealing with depression. You may need medication. You may find that support groups help. Most major cancer-treatment centers employ therapists who routinely meet with cancer patients. In addition, online and telephone help are available.

Recognize that although periods of sadness and depression are a normal part of the grieving process, getting stuck in long-term depression is counterproductive. Norman Cousins, the late editor of the *Saturday Review*, believed that depression was as much an enemy as the cancer. During his illness, he rented every comedy videotape he could find, and he credited laughing with a large part of his successful treatment.

It used to be that a diagnosis of cancer was a death sentence. This is no longer true. Get busy doing what you need to do. You need to get cracking with your life. Your research (like reading this book) will lead you to all the things you can do to increase your odds, to take control, and to help you maintain a decent quality of life. You have, by this time, settled on a treatment. That's a big step toward beating your disease.

Join a support group. Your hospital probably sponsors one. If it doesn't have a prostate-specific group, it may offer general cancer-support sessions. There are also wonderful national groups available (See the "List of Support Groups" on page 80).

Form your own personal support group. I was extremely fortunate. My wife watched for my mood swings and got me talking about what was going on. This was a great help. As a bonus, I never had to ask my friends for support. They immediately rallied around and manifested their support in many ways. Some arrived with books and articles. Some called regularly to make sure I was okay. Some ran errands, cooked food, sent cookies, offered financial support, offered rides—anything they could think of that might be helpful. Others wrote letters giving moral support.

Don't be shy. If your friends don't automatically approach you with offers of help, take it upon yourself to approach them. Do it individually, or call a meeting. Tell them you are enlisting their aid on your support team. Ask them if they will accept assignments. Your friends may feel helpless to know how to aid you, so they may eagerly embrace the chores you assign. Write down a list of your friends, and work from that list to make assignments. Ask for company and a ride to the blood-donor center when you give blood; you may not feel up to driving home alone afterward. Ask a friend to be administrator of your living will, and say why you have picked him or her for the job. The responses of your friends will surprise and delight you.

Some people will be very put off by your illness. Some years ago, I received a call from a friend who had moved across the country. He told me he had developed asbestosis and the doctors gave him no chance of recovery. I expressed my regret to him, but I was paralyzed at the prospect of his death. I simply had no idea what to do for him, and I regret to this day that I failed to think of any way to get past my block and face his problem in the helpful way that so many of my friends did for me.

One of the ways you can help yourself—and your friends—is to let them know *how* to help you. They, like you, feel uncomfortable with the disease, and they don't know what to do with their feelings. Knowing what to do to help will make them feel better—and help you rally the support you need. Neighbors stopped me to volunteer to donate blood if I needed it. They wanted to express their support in a concrete way. If you can't think of a way a friend might help you, ask if he or she would be willing to donate blood should you need it. You probably won't need it, but the donor will feel a part of your team, will keep tabs on you, and may find other ways to be helpful.

My friends were extraordinary in their caring and aid. The few from whom I asked for specific help were all happy to be involved, and our friendships deepened as a result.

Finally, to deal with depression, there is a certain attitude that I suggest you aim for; if you can achieve this frame of mind, it will enrich the rest of your life. While I was convalescing from my operation, I attended a concert. I reflected that if I had died from my cancer, I would not have been there for that event. The sensuous joy that welled up in me was an amazing experience. Since that night, my depth of enjoyment in even simple things has resulted as an unexpected gift.

My psychologist friend, herself a cancer survivor, conducts breast-cancer support groups. She suggests that people take just such an opportunity each day. Find something beautiful: a flower, a photo of a grandchild, a piece of music. Even while you are doing something mundane like washing the dishes, focus on the beauty in the task and the fact that you are here to enjoy it. I suggest you make this a regular exercise. Look at the flower and revel in the fact that you are here to enjoy it on this wonderful day!

Your first line of support should be your local hospital. Most offer general cancer-support groups. The resources listed here are specific to prostate cancer. They can help in areas that will be most pressing for you and that general support groups won't cover—help, for example, in making your initial treatment choice and later for providing information and support for incontinence and erectile-dysfunction issues.

Us Too!

Website: www.ustoo.com

An independent network of support-group chapters for men with prostate cancer and their families, Us Too! groups offer fellowship, peer counseling, education about treatment options, and discussion of medical alternatives without bias. Get on its e-mail list to receive frequent e-mails about the latest prostate-cancer news.

Man-to-Man

Website: www.cancer.org/m2m/m2mgroup.html

This website lists support groups you can join and describes its individual mentor program.

Don Cooley's Patients Helping Patients (PHP) Subscription Lists

Website: www.cooleyville.com/master/maindiv.htm

Don Cooley is a prostate-cancer survivor. He started an Internet subscription list as a helpful and effective way for prostate patients to communicate with one another. Once you have subscribed to a list, you can read and respond to the messages posted by other members, and other members can read and respond to the messages posted by you. It is a good way to ask questions about a variety of issues regarding your disease and its treatment.

Phoenix5

Website: www.phoenix5.org

While not specifically a support group, this website offers straight answers about topics rarely discussed elsewhere, particularly sexuality issues. It also contains a pretty good glossary.

Cancer Hope Network

Website: www.cancerhopenetwork.org

(877) HOPE-NET

This site will match you with carefully chosen volunteers who will communicate with you on a one-to-one basis. Such contact is helpful in answering questions and provides a means by which you can measure your progress against the experience of others.

CHAPTER 11

The Operation

"Do I Have to Shave?"

The night before your operation, you'll be kept busy. There are two major jobs to perform. The first is to clean out your system. The second is to pump yourself full of antibiotics. Your doctor will give you the drill, and, yes, you'll follow his instructions to the letter! You may have to do things that are unpleasant, but you'll want to give yourself as much help as possible.

You will probably be told not to consume anything but clear liquids (water, apple juice, tea) after 3:00 P.M. or so the day before your operation. You can usually drink clear liquids until midnight, then nothing. Thereafter, you will most likely be instructed to take milk of magnesia and an enema or two. You already know the drill from your biopsy procedure.

My doctor prescribed massive doses of two antibiotics. I had never had a reaction to antibiotics before, but this time was different. I sure got sick from one of those babies. My wife drove me to the hospital at 3:00 in the morning, so that the emergency room folks could stabilize me before my 6:30 A.M. report time.

The only advice I can give regarding this preparation period is to follow instructions. If you know that you have a reaction to certain antibiotics, discuss it with your doctor ahead of time.

By now, you will have signed many papers, but the best is yet to come. As instructed, I had left all my valuables at home, and at the hospital I left my wallet, clothes, keys, and glasses with my wife.

In the pre-op care unit of the hospital, I was asked to undress and get into a hospital smock and cap. The nurse took my temperature, pulse, and blood pressure. I was again asked the usual questions about allergies, what I had eaten, and any other problems. I was asked if I had any dentures, and I was told to urinate.

I was now nervously waiting to be wheeled into the operating room on the gurney. An IV was started, and sensors were applied to my arm and chest. At this point, an intern handed me a clipboard with three pages attached. "Read this and sign it," he instructed. "Gee, Doc. I don't have my glasses with me," I informed him. "In that case," he replied, "I'll have to read it to you"—and he began to read the entire document, starting with something like, "I realize that this procedure might lead to my death. . . . "

I interrupted him halfway through, explaining that I knew that the hospital had to inform me of all the possible complications for liability reasons, and that I was ready to sign. Still, he insisted on reading me the entire document.

This was not exactly a relaxing procedure, but, frankly, it was kind of bizarre and funny, so it failed to bother me much. In facing prostate cancer, I was certainly not ready to give up the fight. I was not ready to die. On the other hand, I had led a good life, and, hell, if I had to die, what better way to do it than while totally and blissfully asleep on the operating table.

The room is kept quite cool, and if they don't offer you a blanket, request one. You will probably get a visit from your surgeon or a member of his staff. During these visits the doctor is invariably cheery. After all, he's at the blunt end of the scalpel. He will leave you to go scrub for the operation.

If you are uncomfortable or start to panic while waiting to go into the operating room, tell the nurse. They can give you a sedative or simply chat with you while you wait. Some hospitals will even play music for you. Keep in mind that just the act of discussing your fear will help. This is also the time when I put my relaxation techniques to good use.

The surgeon needs the area on which he is operating to be free of hair and sterile, so a shave is in order. Your pubic hair will be clipped short and then shaved, as will the hair on your lower abdomen. You may get your shave in the pre-op room, or you may first be wheeled into the operating room. A very impersonal attendant usually does the shaving. Yes, it is a bit embarrassing, but under the circumstances you will not get an erection, and it is over in a minute or two. If you are very lucky, as I was, it will be done while you are asleep, sometimes by the surgeon.

At some point, you may be hooked up to an intravenous bottle. The anesthesiologist may inject a little something into the tube that will put you to sleep before you even get wheeled into the operating room. For that reason, at some hospitals, you will never see the operating room. In others, you will be awake while the surgical staff, gowned and masked, bustles around you.

A blood-pressure cuff will be attached to your arm, and a safety belt will be placed over your knees. In some hospitals, you can have your choice of music playing. If you are still awake, this is another good time to practice your relaxation exercises.

You will be surprised at the number of people present. I think I counted three nurses, two surgeons, and an anesthesiologist.

At some point, a plastic mask will be put over your nose and mouth, and you will be asked to breathe deeply. This was not a particularly uncomfortable procedure, and after a few breaths I was quite out of it.

I do not remember even dreaming during the three hours I was in the operating room. I do remember a nurse talking to me in the recovery room and the quite pleasant feeling of waking up fully rested.

POST-OP PROTOCOL

In the postanesthetic care unit (recovery room), I soon realized I was not alone. It was a large room with about ten other groggy patients in direct view of the nursing staff. The place was noisy and busy. Someone or something kept squeezing my legs, and there were all kinds of gizmos and tubes attached to all parts of my body. Let's take a quick tour of these contraptions so you'll know what to expect.

Your legs will be encased in bootlike pillows that periodically inflate to squeeze your legs, sort of like a milking machine. This ensures that the circulation in your extremities is stimulated enough to prevent the formation of blood clots.

Moving upward, next is the catheter. You doctor will probably hook you up to this instrument while you are asleep. The tube goes through your penis and into your bladder. At the other end of the tube, hanging below the mattress, is a plastic bag. You will have no urinary control for a while after the operation, and you will be dependent upon this apparatus for two to four weeks. For now, the nurses will take care of the maintenance, for the bag needs to be emptied several times a day.

The big fear most men have is that the catheter tube will slip out of the penis. Do not worry; a little balloonlike contraption inside prevents this. While the nurse is emptying the bag, he or she is also checking the volume and color of the urine. Be prepared for it to be quite red for at least a few days. It is not uncommon for the urine to be somewhat bloody for a week or more. After you get home, the visiting nurses will also monitor the color of your urine.

Poking out from somewhere in your abdomen will probably be a little plastic spout. This permits drainage of your wounds. It feels strange to have an alien piece of pipe sticking out of you, but there is normally no pain or discomfort associated with this contraption. At some point before you leave the hospital, it will be removed and the small hole will be closed with stitches that were already placed there when the drainage spout was first created. There is little discomfort with this procedure, which takes only a second or two.

Farther up on your body, you may find yourself hooked up to a gizmo that monitors your vital signs. A blood-pressure cuff on your arm may automatically inflate, and sensors may monitor your heart activity. In some hospitals, monitoring is instead done manually on a periodic basis. There is no pain associated with this, and the minor annoyance of being poked and prodded is ameliorated by the fact that it breaks the boredom.

The intravenous bottle, which was attached to you earlier, is still attached and dripping merrily away.

A clip may be attached to your finger to monitor the oxygen in your blood. Your temperature may be taken in your ear with a tympanic-membrane thermometer. A cardiac monitor will be beeping softly.

You may be on oxygen for a while. This is usually administered through lightweight tubes that run over your ears and deliver the air directly into your nostrils. This device is no more annoying than a pair of reading glasses.

A nurse will probably come around at half-hour intervals to do some exercises that are important in helping you recover from your operation. I had been briefed on these at my pre-op testing session, so I knew to also do them once I'd been moved to my own room. In my case, the first exercise was to inhale deeply, hold my breath for two seconds, and then exhale. I repeated this a couple of times.

The next exercise was to inhale and then cough deeply. I was instructed to bend my knees a bit and to hold my hand over the incision area to relieve the strain. After this, I was asked to turn gently from side to side.

The final exercise involved pointing my toes toward the foot of the bed, then relaxing them. Next, I flexed my toes toward my head and then relaxed. Finally, I circled both ankles to the left and right. I repeated this drill three times, then rested for five minutes or so before repeating.

After the operation, the surgeon visited my wife in the waiting room and informed her of my progress. About an hour later I was on my way to my assigned room—and an emotional meeting with my wife. It was good to be alive, even though I had all sorts of tubes coming out of me. If you have no wife or special partner in your life, ask a good friend to meet you in your room to celebrate the fact that you've made it through this difficult stage of your recovery from cancer.

CHAPTER 12

The Hospital Stay

"Who Are All These People?"

You have just undergone an operation that doctors consider one of the more difficult ones. Your prostate has been removed, and probably, as a protective measure, your lymph nodes as well.

You will not be particularly hungry, but do try to drink some broth or juice. Jello is another treat that goes down particularly well.

There are two areas of hospital service that are ripe for mistakes. Don't take a pill without knowing its name and its purpose. Also, be sure to check the food you are served, especially if you have dietary restrictions. Hospital food service has improved greatly over the years; in some facilities, you can even select your next several meals from a menu with limited but not unappetizing options. Still, be sure to check what you are served.

I was offered two or three alternatives for each meal. Each day, the patient-care assistant collected the card where I'd indicated my choices, and I was served what I ordered at least 95 percent of the time. At any rate, if you have a choice during your first day or two, stick with the lighter fare. Let the surf and turf wait for later, when your gastrointestinal tract settles down.

Most hospitals now post in each room a document listing patient rights and responsibilities. Even if your hospital doesn't post such a document, you have certain rights, and if you are smart, you will observe certain rules of conduct as a good patient. The list of "Patient Rights and Responsibilities" on pages 86–87 is a compilation of several documents I have read, but it follows generally the Jefferson Medical System list at the Bryn Mawr Hospital.

- Under any circumstances, you have the right to medical care and services without discrimination based on race, color, sex, sexual preference, religion, national origin, or source of payment.

- You have the right to formulate and prepare an advance directive and to have that directive followed to the letter.

- You have the right and the responsibility to know which hospital rules and regulations affect you. If you are asked to do something you don't agree with, ask by whose authority you are required to do so.

- You are certainly entitled to respectful, quality care given by trained personnel with high professional standards that are maintained and reviewed.

- You have the right to expect that your designated doctor, and not an intern or resident, will be presiding over your care.

- You have the right and the duty to insist that you, or a responsible person designated by you, be informed in terms you can understand of everything done to and for you. This includes information about your diagnosis, treatment, medication, and prognosis.

- You have the right to be told about any research programs that might pertain to your disease. (There are certain rights connected with clinical trials; these are further discussed in Chapter 15.)

- Except in the case of emergencies, you have the right to give or decline your informed consent before the start of any procedure or treatment. Indeed, your physician is required to obtain such consent before proceeding.

- You have the right to medical privacy. Discussion of your case, examination, treatment, consultation, and finances should be held as confidential—and handled discreetly.

- You have the right to refuse any treatment, drugs, or procedures offered, to the extent permitted by law. If you do so, a physician should inform you of the medical consequences of your refusal.

- You have the right to go to another facility. The receiving facility must first agree to accept you. In addition, you or your delegated representative must have received complete information about the needs for, consequences of, and alternatives to such a transfer.

- You have the right to an interpreter, if needed and available.

- You should have access to all records pertaining to your treatment, unless the attending physician specifically prohibits such information for good medical reasons.

- You have the right to see your bills and have them explained to you, and you should, upon request, receive information and counseling on the availability of known financial resources for your health care.

- You have the right to be informed of the mechanisms for settling disputes and grievances.

- Good common sense should tell you that there are behaviors and procedures for which you as a patient are responsible. You should show consideration for other patients and hospital staff by controlling noise, keeping your visitors under control, and refraining from smoking.

- You are responsible for providing complete information about your previous illnesses, medication, and medical history.

- You are responsible for following the medical orders and instructions of your hospital care givers. If you disagree with any of those orders, you are responsible for letting them know that you disagree. You are then responsible for following the procedures for resolving such disputes.

- You are a damned fool if you consume alcoholic beverages or drugs during your hospital stay without your doctors' permission. Such behavior can compromise the effects of your treatment.

- You should be prepared to assume financial responsibility for payment for services. If you will be unable to pay your bill, you are responsible for notifying the hospital in advance. Sit down with the designated personnel to work out an agreeable arrangement.

- You should not wander away from the area to which you are assigned. If you do leave the area, do so only with permission and with the knowledge of personnel on duty as to where you will be and how long you will be gone.

- Remember the PITA rule, namely, that pains-in-the-ass get begrudging service. Your hospital crew works hard and is frequently overworked. The crewmembers are not hired to cater to your every whim. Treat them with patience and respect, and your care will improve in direct proportion.

Space for Your Notes:

....

....

....

....

....

....

....

THE HOSPITAL STAFF

This is a good time to introduce you to the staff in charge of your rather beat-up bod. In some hospitals, you will see only a nurse and a doctor. This is particularly true of small community hospitals. As health-care costs have skyrocketed, larger hospitals have tried to use their labor more efficiently, giving rise to a whole hierarchy of practitioners.

The following is a general list of the people you may encounter at the hospital. Again, remember that each facility is organized in its own way. A worksheet that follows provides space for you to write down the names and titles of the individuals on your health-care team, as well as how to reach them.

Attending Physician: This is your doctor. He or she is probably the one who operated on you. He and his colleagues are responsible for the overall supervision of your treatment. This is the person who signs off on all tests, treatments, and medications.

Consultants: These are specialists in various areas who check on you at the request of your attending physician.

Interns: These overworked doctors have finished medical school and are serving a one- or two-year apprenticeship before getting their license to practice.

Residents: These doctors have completed their internship and are licensed to practice medicine. They are here to learn a specialty. Most of the residents you will meet are M.D.s who are studying urology, surgery, or oncology.

Fellows: These doctors have gone through medical school and have completed one or two years learning a subspecialty. Generally, the fellows you meet will be interested in urological surgery.

Medical Students: If you are in a teaching hospital, typically one associated with a medical school, you may be visited by a delegation on "rounds." A senior doctor will be accompanied by a horde (it seems) of medical students. Though you may feel like a specimen (which you are), you can gain some satisfaction from knowing that you are a vital link in the medical progress. It is also typical in teaching hospitals for senior medical students to drop in from time to time to talk briefly with you, monitor your vital signs, and the like. This may be somewhat annoying, but it does serve a purpose other than to advance the students' training. In these days of staff shortages, anyone monitoring your progress with educated eyes may catch a problem that others are too busy to spot.

Registered Nurses (RNs): Your care and comfort for the two to four days following your surgery will be determined by these hard workers. More so than your doctor, they keep watch over you, dispense medication, carry out your doctor's orders, relieve discomfort or pain, and monitor your progress. They will also teach you how to take care of yourself after you leave the hospital.

Patient-Care Technicians (PCTs): Working under the direct supervision of your RN, a PCT is responsible for taking your temperature and blood pressure, drawing blood for tests, taking electrocardiograms, helping get you ambulatory, helping you shave, providing for your personal cleanliness, and getting you out of the hospital comfortably.

Patient-Care Assistants (PCAs): The PCA is the one who cleans your room and delivers your food. If you are cold or uncomfortable, the PCA will deliver extra pillows or blankets.

Licensed Practical Nurses (LPNs): These folks perform many of the duties of the PCT and some of the duties of the RN. If you need someone in your room with you around the clock, it may be a LPN who can assess any emergency and get the proper relief or help.

Physician's Assistants (PAs): Physician's assistants have a college degree and two years of health profession training. They must undergo an examination to be certified and licensed by the state.

Social Workers: Social workers assist you and your family in planning for your discharge and for any psychological and social problems that may arise.

Student Nurses: These are nurses in training from the local colleges, universities, and teaching hospitals.

Candy Stripers: Candy stripers are volunteers who run errands for the staff, generally make themselves useful, and help cheer up the place.

Home-Care Coordinators: They will help you arrange for visiting nurses, as well as for other professional services to be provided once you get home. If special equipment is required, they'll arrange for that, too.

Diagnostic Staff: These are technicians who perform any diagnostic tests your doctor may require. These could include such things as blood tests and X rays.

Therapists: You probably won't need one of these professionals, but if you need aid in your recovery process, they are trained to help. Various therapists help stroke victims, for example. Occupational therapists teach ADL (activities of daily living): feeding oneself, brushing teeth, etc. Physical therapists help exercise one's various body parts.

Chaplains: In some hospitals, the friendly staff chaplain may visit you. I am not very observant religiously, but I was deeply moved by the visit of the hospital chaplain. This was a gentle reminder that there is a rich spiritual side to life and that it is a blessing to acknowledge your gratitude for life and the healing process.

Hospice Staff: In the event that you are terminally ill, these folks are trained to provide much needed and welcome physical, emotional, and spiritual care. Dying is, after all, something we all must experience. We are helped into this world. How wonderful it is that we can now find help when we are ready to leave it.

Nutritionists: These folks are trained to help you formulate a plan for eating in the most beneficial way, given the facts of your illness and progress. (It might be wise to consult one before your treatment.) Be sure to inform your nutritionist of any previous problems that might affect your diet. Diabetes, food allergies, and personal preferences all play an important role in what will be suggested.

Visiting Nurses: With the advent of "managed care," hospitals are constrained to get you home as quickly as possible. Once there, you will still need some attention and monitoring of your progress. Someone must look out for danger signals in your convalescent period. In many cases it will be a visiting nurse or a nurse from the local hospital's outreach nursing group. In my case, the visiting nurses proved to be highly caring, knowledgeable, helpful people. Continue to use your notebook, and write down any questions you might have for your nurse. (The role of the visiting nurse is further described in Chapter 13.)

LIST OF HEALTH-CARE PROVIDERS

Name	Position	How reached?

Space for Your Notes:

THE RECOVERY STAGE: WALKING, EATING, AND GETTING BACK TO NORMAL

During World War II, many field hospitals came under enemy attack. When that happened, it was necessary to move wounded soldiers to the air-raid shelters. It was quickly discovered that walking, even directly following an operation, speeded the recovery rate of surgery patients.

Based on this and subsequent experience, it will be early in your recovery that your patient-care technician will invite you to take a walk. You won't feel much like walking, but do it anyway. It is a bit of a production. In my case, the PCT helped me sit up and get into a gown. Then he took my urine bag and tied it to an IV stand on wheels. He helped me stand up, and I leaned on the IV stand, pushing it with me as we walked down the hall. It wasn't too bad, though I did get very tired after going only halfway down the hall. He helped me back into bed.

I was accompanied on one more jaunt, longer this time, and by the third time, I was able to get up and out of bed by myself. On my first solo trip I only walked back and forth in my room, but after that I felt comfortable enough to venture out.

There was relatively little pain or discomfort involved in this process, though it did take some doing. Fatigue was more of a problem. The importance of walking was emphasized both in the hospital and at home afterwards. I enjoyed a good feeling of accomplishment when I kept at it, and I rapidly regained strength.

During the remainder of my hospital stay, the oxygen tube was removed, as was the drain. I was slowly weaned to more solid food. It takes a while for the alimentary canal to return to full function after major surgery, and your caregivers will probably want you to have a bowel movement before you leave the hospital. In order to facilitate a normal bowel movement without strain, you will probably be given stool softeners. My movements remained erratic well into my recovery.

The doctor reported that my prostate gland had been one of the largest in the hospital's history. Additionally, the pathological examination of the removed gland revealed that my cancer was even more dangerous than the original Gleason grade had indicated. The tumors turned out to be a Gleason 7. I felt very relieved that I had decided to have the damned thing removed.

LEAVING THE HOSPITAL

The doctor credited my rapid recovery from the surgery to my walking, and I was allowed to go home on the third day. First, though, the nurse went over important procedures that I needed to follow at home. (These are reviewed in the next two chapters.) They included personal cleanliness, the importance of walking, and conditions to watch for (fever, wound infection, etc.). She instructed me and my wife on the use of the catheter, hooked me up to a day bag (described on pages 95–96), and gave us a complete set of day and night bags to take with us. She went over the prescriptions that the doctor had written for me and told me how to take them.

Among the prescriptions were a few to be taken optionally in case of discomfort. I was thrilled that I was subsequently able to manage my pain with the use of Tylenol alone. She handed me a strong pain reliever to take if I had discomfort on the way home, gave me a touching peck on the cheek, and turned me over to the PCT, who wheeled me to my car. It's strange that after prompting you to walk as much as you can, they wheel you out of the hospital. (I guess they don't want anything to happen to you until you're safely out of their jurisdiction.)

I would be disallowed from driving for a few weeks. This was not only because the incision needed time to heal. The fear was that I might suddenly have to slam on the brakes, and the resultant pain might make me cause an accident. I would just have to be chauffeured for a while. I was also told to avoid lifting anything heavier than a book.

I did feel every bump in the road on the way home, but I was happy to be out of the hospital and alive. The scenery was delicious!

Space for Your Notes:

CHAPTER 13

Maintenance

"What Is That Strange Thing Between My Legs?"

The prostate gland completely surrounds the urethra, the vessel that carries urine away from the bladder. In the course of the operation, the urethra is stretched. This may cause the penis to pull into the sack of the scrotum. Your testicles are also enlarged, and a lot of abdominal fat drops down as a result of the operation. Between the swelling, the pulling, and the fat, my penis completely disappeared. I was left with a tube coming out of my scrotum. Yipes! On good days, I could see the head sticking out. This is a common problem, but one that is rarely discussed. See the Phoenix5 website at www.phoenix5.org for helpful information on **penis retraction**.

It is important to keep everything clean. I took showers (baths were not advised) with my night bag resting on the floor outside the shower. To prevent infection, you must clean around the penis. This means poking around inside the scrotum for the retracted penis, a process that takes some getting used to. At the time, I failed to realize that the catheter was securely anchored, so I proceeded kind of cautiously and tentatively. Later, I became bolder. Although doing what's necessary to keep the area clean feels and looks strange, it is actually easily accomplished. You won't hurt anything, and maintaining proper hygiene will save you much trouble.

The management of the catheter is a bit harder. Your nurse will go over the procedure, but I will review it here as a reminder. There are several parts to the apparatus. A tube comes from the bladder and passes through the urethra, exiting at the tip of the penis. An adhesive bandage or velcro fastener secures the tube to the thigh while allowing enough leeway so that you can move comfortably. The other end of the tube goes into a rubberlike bag that acts as a reservoir for the urine.

You use two bags alternately. Both have spouts at the bottom for emptying. The larger bag is the night bag; it will hold an entire night's output. This is hung lower than the top of the mattress so that gravity helps urine flow into the bag. On some models, a clamp on the tube secures it to the bed linens.

In the morning, you unhook and unclamp the bag, empty it into the toilet, and change to the day bag. This one is long and thin, with two straps. You disconnect the tube going into the night bag, insert it into the top of the day bag, and strap the bag to your thigh or over your knee. The bag is thin enough that you can wear it under loose-fitting pants. I wore jogging pants with snaps down the side. When I needed to empty the bag, I unsnapped the side of the pants, leaned my knee on the toilet, and opened the faucet. This made the often-required task a lot easier.

After each bag is used, it should be flushed thoroughly with water and the valves swabbed with alcohol. It is then hung up to dry. Similarly, the fitting on the new bag should be swabbed before you attach the hose. In the evening, you reverse the process, switching to the night bag before going to bed.

The first couple of times I made the switch, my wife stood by to lend a hand. After a few tries, I was able to do it alone. This was the most troublesome problem of the entire battle. It does serve to keep you close to home. A few of my buddies went out to restaurants with the contraption completely and discretely hidden, but they too felt that wearing the catheter was far more debilitating than the operation itself.

The day bag really can be hidden under regular clothing, but a full bag has some weight to it, so if you venture out, be sure to know where there are places the bag can be emptied. To me, it felt as though I were dragging around a ball and chain, and I was nervous about the whole business. As a result, I stayed close to home, just going out for increasingly longer walks. As it turned out, I only used the catheter for two weeks, though some of my cancer buddies had it on for three to four weeks. It wasn't a huge price to pay for extending my life.

Today, they get you out of the hospital as quickly as possible. This is not necessarily a bad thing. Before leaving, I was visited by a social worker on the staff of my urologist. She checked to make sure I understood my prescriptions and how I was to behave, and she had answers to any remaining questions. She also arranged for nurses to visit me at home and set up an appointment two weeks later with my urologist.

The day after I returned home, I was visited by a nurse from my local hospital. (Even though I had not chosen that hospital for my operation, it was the one located nearest to my house, so it's where the visiting nurses came from.) She had the complete history of my case and indicated she would be visiting every other day for a while. She took my temperature and blood pressure and then asked a dozen questions or so: Was I eating properly? How was my appetite? What medication was I taking? Was I experiencing pain?

She inquired as to the frequency of my bowel movements, reminding me not to strain for the next week or two. She instructed me on the use of over-the-counter stool softeners.

She then checked to see that my catheter was performing properly and noted the color of the urine. She gave me instructions to call her office if I noticed any problems, if my temperature increased significantly, or if I had any questions at all. She then took me for a walk. A neighbor spotted me and slammed on his brakes, jumped out of his car, and came to congratulate me. "I heard they had you old folks up and around quickly, but this sure is something," he joked. By the time I was finished with my visiting nurse some two weeks later, she was walking this same neighbor down the street after an unexpected bypass operation.

I ran a low-grade fever for more than a week after the operation. The nurse monitored the temperature fluctuations but said they were nothing to be concerned about. I had many questions that she patiently answered. By now, any modesty I might have had was gone, and I was left with great admiration for these comforting and professional angels of mercy.

I can't stress enough the importance of good nursing care. My doctor was with me for the three hours of my operation and for office visits afterwards. He was absolutely great. But it was the nurses who spent long hours tending to my care and well-being. The depth of their knowledge astonished me.

Several maintenance issues will arise during this period. You need to keep the incision area clean, but regular baths are prohibited. Sponge baths or showers are usually prescribed for the first week or two after the operation. The plastic strips over your incision will normally start to peel off by themselves in about ten days. If in doubt about any of this, call your nurse.

I think I feared the removal of the catheter more than I feared the surgery. On the other hand, I reasoned that my doctor had used such a gentle touch during the digital exam, it might not be so bad. So I was a bit nonplussed when I returned two weeks after my operation and was turned over to a technician to remove the catheter.

She had me lower my pants and lie back on the table. She explained that she was deflating the balloonlike thing that kept the tube in, and it would take just a minute. I felt nothing during this part of the procedure. She then told me to take a deep breath and hold it. I inhaled, felt a quick sort of tickle in my penis, and she said, "Done," before I could hold my breath. I felt no pain. What a relief!

I am told that this experience is the rule, with very few exceptions. Only one of my buddies had pain with the catheter removal, so it is possible, but apparently the anticipation is worse than the actual event.

The nurse said to expect a period of urinary incontinence. **Kegel exercises** were recommended to build up the strength of the sphincter muscles that control the urine. These consist of tightening the sphincter muscles without tightening the abdomen. The advantage of doing Kegels is that you can do them any time, anywhere—at your desk, at a movie, at the dinner table.

For some reason, I had trouble isolating the muscles and keeping them contracted. The best advice came from one of the nurses. "Pretend," she advised, "that you are at a dinner party and feel the need to pass wind. Now hold it in. Those are the muscles you need to strengthen." Her advice helped, but long after the warning tingles stopped, I found that I had most of my accidents when I had to pass wind (being an "old fart," this happened frequently). I never had a bad accident; most of my incidents involved only a drop or two, with an occasional short squirt. (See page 101 for more information on Kegel exercises.)

After this instruction, the doctor came in to answer any further questions, and then I walked out, finally free of pipes and tubes. Having been forewarned about leakage, I had come to my catheter-removal appointment with pads for protection (see pages 99–100 for information about pads).

CHAPTER 14

Incontinence and Impotence

"Am I Destined for Pads and Viagra?"

INCONTINENCE

The joke is, "If you take Viagra for impotence, what do you take for incontinence?" The answer is "Niagara." What is no joke is the possibility that your postoperative incontinence might become permanent.

Protection comes in three basic forms, all of which are found in the incontinence-supplies section of most pharmacies and some supermarkets. Each of the three basic configurations may also come in various levels of absorbency. You will see from the ready availability of these products that you have plenty of company.

Full absorbent pants and briefs are sized briefs that are lined with an absorbent substance. They have elastic around the legs and waist that keep the moisture in. They are the most absorbent of the three general styles, but they are bulky, necessitating loose-fitting clothing. They may be your best choice for night use, at least in the beginning.

The belted undergarment is a large, absorbent rectangle, usually sold with two elastic bands that are buttoned into the tops of the product. When worn, it looks like a diaper with two belts of elastic at the waist on each side. These, too, come in various levels of absorbency, so shop carefully. This product is much less bulky and is more comfortable to wear. Since these are not sized or truly shaped, they do tend to bunch up, particularly between the legs. I often felt like someone was squeezing my testicles, necessitating a visit to the nearest private room for an adjustment.

Guards, also called pads or shields, are the most comfortable to wear. Typically, the pad is about two to three inches wide, with a strip of paper-covered adhesive running lengthwise down the pad. You strip off the paper and press the pad into your brief-type shorts (these don't work with boxer shorts). The adhesive helps keep the pad in place. These, too, come in several absorbencies; they are the least effective of the three styles, but the most comfortable. I found that if I placed the front (indicated by an arrow on some products) just under the waistband of my briefs, the pad fell into the most comfortable position for me.

I quickly found that I was most continent at night. I therefore opted, in the beginning, for the belted undergarment. Before long, I was spending the night totally dry, so I switched to regular boxer shorts. These served to catch the few droplets that infrequently spilled during the night.

Of more concern were the so-called stress accidents. When getting in and out of my car, or rising from a chair, I would feel a funny tingle in the tip of my penis, and I knew to run for the nearest bathroom—if I could make it. Here, too, the anticipation proved worse than the actual event. There was rarely more than a small wet spot on the surface of my protection. As a result, I wore the belted undergarment for longer jaunts when I was uncertain of finding a toilet and the more comfortable pad when closer to home.

I found that with any of these alternatives, going to the men's room in a public place was relatively easy. I simply unzipped as usual, reached in with my left thumb and pulled down the waistband of my briefs, and then found and aimed my penis with the other hand. You might want to practice this at home before venturing out. Once the catheter came out, I experienced steady improvement in the strength of my urine stream (you'll be asked about that), but the urine pretty much shot out in random directions. This is a common problem, as is retraction of the penis. (See the Phoenix5 website at www.phoenix5.org for more information on these matters.)

Several other recommendations exist that may help with incontinence. Each of these suggestions has its critics, so check with your doctor or nurse to see what they recommend.

Some suggest that you attempt to stop the flow momentarily while urinating, since to do so exercises the urinary sphincter muscles that have been weakened. Others say this is counterproductive. Most doctors suggest that you drink two quarts of liquid a day, a practice that is supposed to get the system functioning again and exercised properly. I found it hard to drink that much and discovered that I could not drink at all after 8:00 P.M. if I wanted to remain dry overnight. If you must attend a meeting or go on a trip, you should limit your fluid consumption prior to the event. All caffeinated beverages, alcoholic drinks, and grapefruit products will make you urinate more often, so avoid them.

The best line of prevention for incontinence is the Kegel exercises mentioned in the last chapter (see page 98 for a description of how to isolate the muscle involved). Here's more information about how to do the exercises: Start with a session of "long" Kegels. Contract the muscle for ten seconds, then relax for eight seconds. Repeat the whole cycle, working up to fifteen times. If you get tired and find that you can no longer control the muscles, stop. Remember that fifteen repetitions is a goal you're working toward. Your endurance will improve with time.

After a cycle of the long Kegels, rest for about half a minute, and then follow with the "fast" Kegels. Squeeze and hold for one second, relax completely for a second, and repeat for a total of five times. Then relax for ten seconds. Do a total of four or five sets of five reps.

Two complete sessions a day—a set of the long and a set of the fast Kegels—are the recommended drill, once when you wake up and once in the early evening. The exercises are invisible to others, so I also tried to squeeze in a midday session while sitting at my desk.

"But What If . . . ?"

What if you can't control your bladder at all? First of all, give it time. A year or possibly two is not all that unusual. Even if after that length of time you're still having problems, all is not lost. In addition to the Kegel exercises, there are several other avenues to explore:

- Consult with your dietician about a diet that will help you retain fluids.

- Your doctor can suggest other solutions that will help get rid of the problem. Several medications have proved effective in helping control urinary incontinence, and biofeedback and electrical stimulation are other alternatives.

- Surgical procedures exist that create artificial sphincters to help control the problem.

I try not to take medication unless it is absolutely necessary. After nine months I was continent at night, but sometimes I dribbled during the day. I decided to stick with the Kegels and the pads, even if I had to live with them forever. I doubt I will have to, but it is a solution that is relatively easy to deal with. It is a small price to pay for being alive.

IMPOTENCE

Okay. You want the whole story on impotence. No holds barred.

None of the treatments for prostate cancer are guaranteed to preserve your ability to have an erection. Every person is different, and the degree of impotency will vary with each individual and with each therapy.

My buddy who opted for hormone therapy said it took a lot of effort to get an erection during treatment. He was rarely in the mood, and if he did ejaculate, there was little or no semen.

External-beam radiation patients report that their sexual function gradually decreases during the course of their therapy. Seed-implant patients report the same problem and also cite lack of interest and fatigue. Cancer patients often experience depression (see Chapter 10) in addition to the physical symptoms. It is difficult to initiate intimate contact when you are feeling nauseated and are fighting cancer.

You should know that you probably won't have an erection for a long while, and maybe never (the "never" part is covered in the "what if" section on pages 103–104). You will be heartened to know that you can still have orgasms—intense ones—without an erection.

The nerve-sparing operation devised by Dr. Walsh is designed to save the nerves that are responsible for erections. Even under the best of circumstances, your reproductive system has undergone a hell of a trauma, so don't expect too much too soon. The removal of the prostate also means that you will not ejaculate semen.

Your doctor will probably prescribe Viagra. Some doctors are prescribing the pill early in the convalescent period, feeling that it speeds up refunctioning. Normally, the pill is taken an hour before you expect to begin lovemaking. However, if plans change and no sexual stimulation occurs once you've taken the medication, you'll experience no effect.

In my case, the 50-mg dose I was given had no effect at all. Neither did the 100-mg dose to which I was switched. My general practitioner recommended that I take one pill before bedtime on the night before I planned to have intercourse, then another dose an hour before. The best I was able to achieve was a halfhearted erection that was not firm enough for insertion.

Fortunately, after forty-seven years of marriage, my wife and I are still very much in love, so there was much we could do to enjoy physical love with each other. We have always spent a good deal of time in foreplay, and the cuddling, massaging, and kissing remained as satisfying as ever, perhaps more so. To give your partner complete satisfaction, you may have to rely on oral and/or hand stimulation to achieve climax.

I was unable to get an erection under any circumstances, but using a vibrator I was able to be stimulated to intense, satisfying orgasms. I was advised to "use it or lose it," so I also self-stimulated, not always to a successful orgasm. I am told that some men never fully recover their ability to have erections, and they leave it at that. After discussing this openly, you and your partner may decide to just enjoy the other alternatives.

My wife and I were unwilling to give up that final pleasurable act, and I felt rather impatient. I was told to give it a year, possibly two. I can't say that it wasn't a frustrating problem for me. Even the hour-before bit removes a good deal of spontaneity from the act.

My frustration was made a lot easier by my wife's open attitude. I urge you to be as open with your mate as you can possibly be. Discuss your feelings. Talk about your frustrations. Be sure to talk about what does feel good when you make love, and give each other lots of hugs and kisses in between.

After nine months and still no success, I was told about the orange-juice trick. If you put a Viagra pill in water, it takes a long time to dissolve. This is because it needs acid to be effective. It was suggested that I break up the pill before swallowing it. You can do this by chewing it, but it tastes bitter. I used a pill splitter (available in most drugstores) to chop it into six or seven pieces. I then swallowed the pieces with some orange juice to supply the necessary acidity. That ploy started me on the road to erectile function.

If you are uncomfortable talking about sex with your partner, I urge that you both go for counseling. Cancer Care (see page 137 in the Resources section) can refer you to a helpful professional in your area. There are positive things you can do, and you may just find that this dialogue brings you closer together. (The worksheet on page 105 may be helpful in getting the discussion started.)

"But What If . . . ?"

If you don't heal completely, and your erectile dysfunction remains unresponsive to Viagra, all is not lost. There are alternatives:

- Suction pumps (**vacuum constriction devices** or VCDs) are one alternative. These are tubes into which the penis is inserted. Suction is then supplied, either by battery operation or by manual pumping. The suction draws blood into the penis, producing an erection. An elastic band is then placed at the base of the penis to keep the blood in the shaft. This will keep the erection for twenty-five minutes or so, but it must be removed after thirty minutes to restore circulation. As with many of these methods, some practice is advised before you incorporate it into your lifestyle. Some couples report great success with the method, and it has the advantage of being a relatively inexpensive solution.

■ Another solution is the **penile suppository**. This is a thin cylinder made of medicated material that is inserted into the penis by means of a plastic device, producing an erection. The suppository dissolves on its own, like a rectal suppository. It sounds icky and painful but usually is easy and painless. The trick is to be sure that you urinate before you insert the suppository, thereby lubricating the urethra. Few problems are reported from the use of this alternative. You will have to keep Sudafed handy—just in case your erection lasts too long, or you experience any other side effects.

■ Several other medicines exist that can be injected into the penis for the same purpose. Erections will last up to an hour. Again, this sounds painful, but in fact it is not at all uncomfortable. One man I interviewed says his wife enjoys giving him the injection, and she is certainly happy with the outcome. Before deciding on this alternative, ask your doctor about reported side effects. They are rare, but the possibility is greater with this method than with the suppository.

■ **Penile implants** are an expensive but viable alternative. In their simpler form, a semirigid rod is implanted in the penis. This is a surgical procedure, with the usual surgical risks. With the implant, the penis is just hard enough to enable penetration. It remains in a drooping position, but can be inserted for intercourse.

■ **Inflatable implants** are a more complex solution. They create more realistic erections in that the implanted cylinders are pumped full of liquid. There are several brands of implants, ranging from expensive to very expensive.

My suggestion is to try the Viagra route first, then work your way up. Of course, discuss all of this with your doctor.

SEX-ISSUES WORKSHEET

Use the following chart to define the sex issues to be discussed with your partner and, if applicable, your therapist.

Until you are able to enjoy intercourse together, you and your partner can decide which of the following intimate activities you enjoy; check them off in the two left-hand columns of the chart below. In the two right-hand columns, check off methods by which you each would be willing to achieve orgasm. Use the blank lines at the bottom of the chart to explore other wishes and desires.

Activity	Yourself	Your Partner	Yourself	Your Partner
Hugging	☐	☐	☐	☐
Kissing	☐	☐	☐	☐
Playacting, fantasizing	☐	☐	☐	☐
Massaging	☐	☐	☐	☐
Showering together	☐	☐	☐	☐
Watching erotic movies	☐	☐	☐	☐
Anal stimulation	☐	☐	☐	☐
Direct hand stimulation	☐	☐	☐	☐
Oral stimulation	☐	☐	☐	☐
Sex toys (e.g., vibrators)	☐	☐	☐	☐
_____	☐	☐	☐	☐
_____	☐	☐	☐	☐
_____	☐	☐	☐	☐
_____	☐	☐	☐	☐
_____	☐	☐	☐	☐

In discussing alternatives, things to consider include:

Just how bothersome is this problem to us?

Are there other ways we can express our love for each other?

How do we feel about the various methods described?

Would either of us mind a penile implant?

How will each of the methods affect the rhythm and atmosphere of our lovemaking?

Space for Your Notes:

CHAPTER 15

Follow-Up and Clinical Trials

"When Do We Celebrate?"

You will get to enjoy many celebrations along the way in this adventure of yours. Each patient and his doctor have their own milestones. I celebrated when I got out of the hospital. I celebrated again when they took the catheter out. But when can you *really* celebrate?

Some doctors say that you will monitor your PSA for the rest of your life, just in case a few bum cells have escaped the envelope and start to spread. Others say that if you get low PSA scores for five years, you are home free.

At this point, you should know the difference between a regular PSA and a sensitive PSA. **Regular PSAs** are given in your urologist's office or at your local hospital. These test results are accurate, but within limits. There is a variant of a few tenths of a point. The tests are not certified to give you a flat 0.0, so that even if the results come out zero, given the plus-or-minus factor for the variant, the results must be given at the high end of the variation. As a result, your flat 0.0 result may come back as 0.3.

There are some labs certified to perform **sensitive PSAs**—that is, to test for the PSA extremely accurately. I live in the Philadelphia area, and the nearest lab for sensitive PSA testing is in New England.

Sending my blood out of the area for testing added a few days of delay in obtaining the results, but it was worth it for the 0.0 result I got back. I have had two such 0.0 results, and I can reasonably conclude that any escaped cells that may exist will probably take a long time to develop, so I can safely celebrate, at least until the next test. (With radiation therapy alone, the PSA drops to an acceptable level, but rarely drops to 0.0.)

"BUT WHAT IF...?"

What if your PSA comes back and shows that you still have cancer cells lurking in your body? If you have had surgery, you can still opt for hormone and/or radiation therapy. If you have only had hormone therapy, you can now opt for surgery. If prostate cancer recurs, follow-up treatment will depend on what treatment you have already undergone, how extensive your cancer is, the grade and stage of the cancer, the site of recurrence, you general health, and your age.

Since each patient is different, consult your doctor for alternatives. If you don't like what he offers, or even if you do, go for a second opinion about the best course of action to take now.

CONSIDERING A CLINICAL TRIAL?

You should know that as of this writing, several new therapies show promise of being cures and/or techniques for treating prostate cancer. A German group has developed a new method of implanting seeds more accurately. For reasons I am unable to fathom, the technique has not been accepted in this country. A highly promising vaccine called **angiostatin** is undergoing Phase II clinical trials in the United States (see the description of the different phases of clinical trials on page 109). This medicine, developed by Dr. Judah Folkman, starves the blood that feeds cancer cells, thereby limiting their growth. Hundreds of other promising treatments are also currently undergoing clinical trials in this country. The Centerwatch website at www.centerwatch.com/patient/studies/CAT36.html lists the many ongoing trials.

If you find yourself contemplating participation in a clinical trial, you need to know just what the procedures will be and what your rights are should you choose to enter the program. Before you can enter a clinical trial, your eligibility—or lack thereof—will be determined. This has nothing to do with how nice a fellow you are. Your medical profile must fit the parameters of the study. Your age, your medical history, and your condition may fail to fit the aims of the research project.

Such research projects are closely monitored and approved by the government. A review board oversees the protocol of each clinical trial, making sure that the risks are as low as possible and determining whether the research is promising enough to justify the cost and effort. The protocol sets out the rules for the trial, the length of the study, how many people will participate, the procedures, the dosages, and the schedule.

When you go to your interview, follow the advice given for your first meeting after diagnosis. (See Chapter 6 and the "Preappointment Worksheet" on page 35.) Take someone with you, take a tape recorder, take a list of questions, and take your notebook. (A list of suggested questions can be found in the "Clinical-Trials Worksheet" at the end of this chapter. Add your own questions to the list and take it with you too.)

Before you enter a study, the researchers will provide you with an **informed-consent document** that tells you about the protocol for the study, stating what will be done, the risks and benefits expected, and how long you will be involved. You should also be informed that you have the right to leave the study at any time. Take the document home with you. Discuss it with your family, your friends, and your doctors. After that, if you decide to sign it, make sure to keep a copy for yourself.

On the one hand, the new protocol may turn out to be the cure for your specific problem. On the other hand, you may be part of a control group. If this is the case, because control-group participants are given placebos that offer no treatment benefit, you can lose valuable time. Find out what happens to patients who are on the placebo after the study is completed. In some cases, the study is relatively short, and if the treatment shows promise, the control group is then put on the medication. During the trial, there is no way to discover whether you are receiving the treatment or the placebo. The double-blind testing procedure ensures that no one you have contact with as a participant knows to which group you belong.

Joining a clinical trial may give you access to treatment that is unavailable to the general public. You will certainly be getting expert care. You will be closely monitored and examined. In addition, you will be contributing to medical progress in a significant way. On the other hand, entering a clinical trial can be extremely time-consuming. There may be side effects or *no* effects. Carefully assess the pros and cons before making your decision. If you do join and find that it is not for you, you can withdraw. It is your moral duty, however, not to withdraw frivolously, and if you do withdraw, to inform the staff of your reasons for leaving the trial.

Be sure to question whether there are any costs to you if you enter the trial, and, if there are, whether your insurance plan will cover the expense. Research costs are not always covered by health plans. Some studies provide a fee to help you cover incidental costs.

Clinical trials are conducted in four stages. **Phase I** trials generally involve only fifty or so patients. The main goals of this phase are to establish safe dosages and to determine whether the treatment causes any harmful side effects. **Phase II** trials typically involve several hundred patients. The treatment's safety is further evaluated and a preliminary assessment is made of the effectiveness of the treatment. **Phase III** trials involve several thousand people. The goal here is to further confirm the safety and efficacy of the treatments and to determine if the treatment can be safely marketed. If the treatment is approved, **Phase IV** studies continue to monitor the safety and effectiveness of the treatment and to discover any long-term side effects. Knowing the facts about a trial will help you make the appropriate decision for you.

It is probably good advice to avoid treatment from a doctor who is sponsoring a clinical trial. This holds true for your second-opinion resource as well. Doctors in this position are naturally hopeful that their trials will show positive results. This disqualifies them from being able to be totally objective in your case.

CLINICAL-TRIALS WORKSHEET

The following questions are those you might want to ask before entering a clinical trial. Many will be answered in the trial's informed-consent document. You may be able to get a copy of that document before your first interview.

What is the purpose of this study? _____

_____

_____

Who is the sponsor? _____

Where will the study be conducted? _____

How much time is involved? _____

How long will the study last? _____

What kinds of procedures are involved? _____

_____

Are hospital stays involved? ☐ Yes ☐ No

How long are the stays? _____

Is the procedure painful? ☐ Yes ☐ No

For how long will I be in pain? _____

Will the study personnel be in contact with my doctor? ☐ Yes ☐ No

Do I continue with my current medications? ☐ Yes ☐ No

What are the benefits of the proposed treatment? _____

_____

What are the risks of the proposed treatment? _____

_____

What are the possible side effects? _____

_____

_____

What other treatment options do I have? _____

_____

What expenses are anticipated? _____

_____

Will I be paid for participating? ☐ Yes ☐ No

Space for Your Notes:

CHAPTER 16

A Final Word

I hope that you feel optimistic and empowered by taking control of your disease. I hope that your experience helps you to survive and, more than that, to live life more fully. Now find an opportunity to go out and help others. It has been clinically proven that those who do have a higher recovery rate.

I'm sure you'll find the support and information you need among the suggested resources in this workbook. If, however, you need further help, and certainly if you have suggestions that would make this workbook more useful, please contact me directly. My e-mail address is newtm@prostateworkbook.com.

I can't promise to answer every e-mail. Fortunately, my life is very busy right now. There is so much I want to do! If I can't answer your question, I will try to pass it on to someone who can. You and I belong to an elite fraternity now, and I hope you'll join the ranks of generous men who have used their experience to help make it easier for others.

Space for Your Notes:

Worksheets for Partners

To the spouse, loved one, or friend of a prostate-cancer patient:

Upon hearing a diagnosis of cancer, your loved one's most probable reactions include panic and shock. At the very least, he is overloaded with new feelings, problems, and decisions to make. Whether you are his spouse, life partner, family member, or trusted friend, you, too, will likely face uncertainty and fear. He has chosen to place his confidence in you as his health-care partner for this crusade. You can be of great help to him—and, not incidentally, to yourself—by becoming a proactive participant in his treatment.

The worksheets and checklists that follow will help you stay focused, which, in turn, will help make his treatment easier to bear. *You* can make the difference between a more comfortable, successful course of treatment and a confusing, second-rate outcome. Read through the material in this book—especially the pointers in Chapter 1 and the worksheets that follow—then roll up your sleeves and pitch in, knowing that you will make a big difference.

Caregivers of the seriously ill have a rough row to hoe. They can use some support themselves. A list of Internet sites offering helpful advice and resources for caregivers appears on page 139.

Worksheets for Partners

Biopsy Results 117

Questions about Testing (3 copies) 118

Preappointment Worksheet 121

Test Records I 122

Post-Testing Questions 123

Test Records II 124

Treatment Option Evaluation 125

Finding a Cancer-Treatment Facility 127

Second-Opinion Questions 128

Treatment Option Evaluation (Second Opinion) 129

Family-Issues Worksheet 131

Blood-Donation Appointments 132

Living-Will Worksheet 133

Preoperative Exam Checklist 134

List of Health-Care Providers 135

BIOPSY RESULTS

Your partner may undergo several biopsies. If you are privy to this information, listen in when the doctor reports. Make sure your partner writes the results in his workbook. If the biopsy is positive, make sure the physician gives you the Gleason score as well. Note it below the chart.

Date	Where performed	Doctor	Results	Doctor's Comments

Space for Your Notes:

QUESTIONS ABOUT TESTING

Your partner will be taking a series of tests. This worksheet helps keep track of them.

What is the name of this test? _____

What is the purpose of this test? _____

_____

Is the test necessary? ☐ Yes ☐ No

Where does he take the test? _____

How long will it take? _____

Will he have to stay overnight? ☐ Yes ☐ No

Will he be able to drive himself home safely after the test? _____

Are there any side effects from the test? ☐ Yes ☐ No

_____

Is there any medication he must take before the test? ☐ Yes ☐ No

_____

Is there any other preparation before the test? ☐ Yes ☐ No Must he fast? ☐ Yes ☐ No

_____

Is there any pain involved in this procedure, and, if so, can he take medication for it? ☐ Yes ☐ No

_____

Would he take the pain medication before the test, or after? _____

When and how does he get the results of the test? _____

_____

Where does he get physical possession of his X rays and plates from any testing?_____

_____

Space for Your Notes:

....

....

....

....

....

....

QUESTIONS ABOUT TESTING

Your partner will be taking a series of tests. This worksheet helps keep track of them.

What is the name of this test? _____

What is the purpose of this test? _____

_____

Is the test necessary? ☐ Yes ☐ No

Where does he take the test? _____

How long will it take? _____

Will he have to stay overnight? ☐ Yes ☐ No

Will he be able to drive himself home safely after the test? _____

Are there any side effects from the test? ☐ Yes ☐ No

_____

Is there any medication he must take before the test? ☐ Yes ☐ No

_____

Is there any other preparation before the test? ☐ Yes ☐ No Must he fast? ☐ Yes ☐ No

_____

Is there any pain involved in this procedure, and, if so, can he take medication for it? ☐ Yes ☐ No

_____

Would he take the pain medication before the test, or after? _____

When and how does he get the results of the test? _____

_____

Where does he get physical possession of his X rays and plates from any testing? _____

_____

Space for Your Notes:

....

....

....

....

....

QUESTIONS ABOUT TESTING

Your partner will be taking a series of tests. This worksheet helps keep track of them.

What is the name of this test? _____

What is the purpose of this test? _____

_____

Is the test necessary? ☐ Yes ☐ No

Where does he take the test? _____

How long will it take? _____

Will he have to stay overnight? ☐ Yes ☐ No

Will he be able to drive himself home safely after the test? _____

Are there any side effects from the test? ☐ Yes ☐ No

_____

Is there any medication he must take before the test? ☐ Yes ☐ No

_____

Is there any other preparation before the test? ☐ Yes ☐ No Must he fast? ☐ Yes ☐ No

_____

Is there any pain involved in this procedure, and, if so, can he take medication for it? ☐ Yes ☐ No

_____

Would he take the pain medication before the test, or after? _____

When and how does he get the results of the test? _____

_____

Where does he get physical possession of his X rays and plates from any testing? _____

_____

Space for Your Notes:

....

....

....

....

....

....

After your partner has undergone all the required tests, his doctor will make an appointment to discuss the results and his treatment alternatives. Check off on the list below what he may need to take to the appointment.

☐ Workbook or applicable worksheets (see Chapter 6)

☐ Pencils, pen

☐ Tape recorder, cassette tape

☐ Location of appointment:_____

  Room #:_____ Time of appointment:_____

☐ Doctor's name: _____

☐ Name of doctor's staff member who made appointment: _____

☐ Doctor's phone number: _____

☐ Insurance cards

  Does doctor accept my partner's insurance? ☐ Yes ☐ No

  If not, what payment is expected at the time of the visit? _____

☐ Credit cards

  Does the doctor accept credit cards? ☐ Yes ☐ No

  Which? _____

☐ General Medical History (see pages 25–29)

☐ List of questions

Space for Your Notes:

....

....

....

....

....

....

....

....

After the testing is done, the results, plates, reports, slides, X rays, etc., need to get to his doctor for his evaluation appointment. If this job falls to you, the following form will help.

Before his appointment:

Step 1: Find out which records his first doctor will need. Place an "X" in the far-left column of the chart below, next to each required item.

Step 2: Write in the current location of that record.

Step 3: If he wants the record(s) sent to his doctor, find out if you can authorize release by phone.

Step 4: Determine when these records will be sent or when they can be picked up.

Step 5: If the office or lab will be sending the records, indicate the name of the person you talked with and how the records will be sent. If you (or your partner) plan to pick them up, check the space in the "Picked up" column when you have them in your possession.

Step 6: If the records will be sent to his doctor, call a few days before his appointment to confirm that they were received. If you have them and are ready to take them with you, check the space in the "Received" column.

X	Records	Location	Phone release okay?	When?	Picked up or sent by	Received
☐	Medical history	Workbook	☐	_____	_____	☐
☐	Biopsy (histology) report	_____	☐	_____	_____	☐
☐	Ultrasound copies	_____	☐	_____	_____	☐
☐	Pathology reports	_____	☐	_____	_____	☐
☐	Pathology slides	_____	☐	_____	_____	☐
☐	X rays	_____	☐	_____	_____	☐
☐	Other	_____	☐	_____	_____	☐
☐	_____	_____	☐	_____	_____	☐
☐	_____	_____	☐	_____	_____	☐

Space for Your Notes:

....

....

After his various tests—such as bone scan, CT scan, and the like—the next appointment is the most vital one your partner will face. The doctor will evaluate the test results and offer suggestions for treatment. Your job is to ask questions of the doctor that your partner forgets to ask and to write down all the comments and answers. Your partner should do the same and compare notes with you later.

What is your assessment of his cancer? _____

What stage would you assign to it? _____

Is it self-contained? ☐ Yes ☐ No

How far has it spread? _____

What other parts of his body are affected? _____

What treatment options are open to him?

☐ Watchful waiting

☐ Hormone therapy

☐ Surgery

☐ Brachytherapy (seeds)

☐ External radiation

☐ Cryosurgery

☐ Other _____

Of the options open to him, what are the various risks? _____

_____

If you were he, which treatment would you choose? _____

_____

Before you leave this appointment, tell the doctor you think it prudent obtain a second opinion and that you want to take all your records with you. (The "Test Records II" worksheet on page 124 will help you make sure you have all of the records you will need.) You might also want to review Chapter 7.

First session notes:

....

....

....

Before you leave the evaluation appointment, check that you have:

☐ Biopsy (histology) report

☐ Ultrasound copies

☐ Pathology reports

☐ Pathology slides

☐ X rays

☐ Other reports or test results

Space for Your Notes:

....

....

....

....

....

....

....

....

....

....

....

....

....

....

....

....

....

....

He must now decide on a treatment. List each treatment option open to him, then write the positive factors of that option on one side of the chart and the negative factors on the other side.

Option: _____

	Positive Factors	**Negative Factors**
Odds of cure:	_____	_____
	_____	_____
Length of treatment:	_____	_____
	_____	_____
Side effects:	_____	_____
	_____	_____
Risks:	_____	_____
	_____	_____
Other factors:	_____	_____

Option: _____

	Positive Factors	**Negative Factors**
Odds of cure:	_____	_____
	_____	_____
Length of treatment:	_____	_____
	_____	_____
Side effects:	_____	_____
	_____	_____
Risks:	_____	_____
	_____	_____
Other factors:	_____	_____

Option: _____

	Positive Factors	Negative Factors
Odds of cure:	_____	_____
	_____	_____
Length of treatment:	_____	_____
	_____	_____
Side effects:	_____	_____
	_____	_____
Risks:	_____	_____
	_____	_____
Other factors:	_____	_____

Option: _____

	Positive Factors	Negative Factors
Odds of cure:	_____	_____
	_____	_____
Length of treatment:	_____	_____
	_____	_____
Side effects:	_____	_____
	_____	_____
Risks:	_____	_____
	_____	_____
Other factors:	_____	_____

FINDING A CANCER-TREATMENT FACILITY

How close is the facility to his home? _____

How many prostate cancer cases does it treat each year? _____

How many prostatectomies does it perform? _____

How many are treated with radiation? _____

What has been its mortality rate? _____

How does that compare with the national average? _____

Does the facility have the ability to do all his testing on-site, including:

☐ Blood work?   ☐ CT scans?   ☐ Bone scans?   ☐ X rays?

What other services does the facility provide?

☐ Nutritionist?   ☐ Cancer support group?   ☐ Psychological help?

☐ Chaplaincy services?   ☐ Social workers?

Other services available: _____

_____

What is the nurse-to-patient ratio? _____

Is care at this facility covered by his health insurance? ☐ Yes ☐ No

What portions and how much of his bill will be covered? _____

_____

What arrangements are available for the payment of the balance? _____

_____

Phone referrals:

National Cancer Institute (free referral services)
(800) 422-6237

American College of Surgeons
(312) 649-7081
Website: www.facs.org

Association of Community Cancer Centers
(301) 984-9496
Website: www.accc-cancer.org

SECOND-OPINION QUESTIONS

After reviewing his records, what is your assessment of his cancer?

What treatment options are open to him?

- ☐ Watchful waiting
- ☐ Hormone therapy
- ☐ Surgery
- ☐ Brachytherapy (seeds)
- ☐ External radiation
- ☐ Cryosurgery

Other options: _____

Of the open options, what are his odds? _____

_____

Of the open options, what are his risks? _____

_____

If you were he, which treatment would you choose? _____

_____

_____

Space for Your Notes:

....

....

....

....

....

....

....

....

....

....

....

(Second Opinion)

He must now decide on a treatment. As you did before, list each treatment option open to him, then write down the positive factors on one side of the chart and the negative factors on the other.

Option: _____

	Positive Factors	**Negative Factors**
Odds of cure:	_____	_____
	_____	_____
Length of treatment:	_____	_____
	_____	_____
Side effects:	_____	_____
	_____	_____
Risks:	_____	_____
	_____	_____
Other factors:	_____	_____

Option: _____

	Positive Factors	**Negative Factors**
Odds of cure:	_____	_____
	_____	_____
Length of treatment:	_____	_____
	_____	_____
Side effects:	_____	_____
	_____	_____
Risks:	_____	_____
	_____	_____
Other factors:	_____	_____

(Second Opinion)

Option: _____

	Positive Factors	**Negative Factors**
Odds of cure:	_____	_____
	_____	_____
Length of treatment:	_____	_____
	_____	_____
Side effects:	_____	_____
	_____	_____
Risks:	_____	_____
	_____	_____
Other factors:	_____	_____

Option: _____

	Positive Factors	**Negative Factors**
Odds of cure:	_____	_____
	_____	_____
Length of treatment:	_____	_____
	_____	_____
Side effects:	_____	_____
	_____	_____
Risks:	_____	_____
	_____	_____
Other factors:	_____	_____

During this appointment with your partner's second-opinion doctor, you may want to review the assessments you made after his first post-testing doctor's appointment (see the first "Treatment Option Evaluation" worksheet on pages 125–126). Does the new doctor agree with your assessment?

Things His Family Might Worry About

Review Chapter 9, then be prepared to answer the following questions as simply as possible, if you are asked:

- Is he in pain?

- Will he die?

- Is it contagious? Will I get it?

- What do the doctors say?

- How is he going to get better?

- Where?

- When?

- Who is the doctor?

- How will he feel after his treatment?

- How long will it take?

- Who is in charge? Name names.

- What other help is he getting?

- Who else knows about this, and how do they feel about it?

- Can we visit him? When?

- How will he feel when we do?

- What does he expect from us?

- How can we help?

BLOOD-DONATION APPOINTMENTS

If your partner opts for surgery and decides to donate blood for his own use during his operation, you can help him keep track of his blood-donation appointments with the following chart.

X	Date	Location	Done
☐	_____	_____	_____
☐	_____	_____	_____
☐	_____	_____	_____
☐	_____	_____	_____
☐	_____	_____	_____
☐	_____	_____	_____

POST–BLOOD DONATION CHECKLIST

☐ Make sure he drinks four extra glasses of nonalchoholic liquids (eight ounces each).

☐ Keep bandage on and dry for five hours after donation.

☐ No heavy exercise or heavy lifting for rest of day.

☐ If he's dizzy, get him to lie down and raise his feet.

☐ If needle site starts to bleed, raise his arm straight up and press the needle-insertion area until the bleeding stops.

☐ He could experience dizziness or weakness. Review his activities to make sure he (and others) are safe under these circumstances.

☐ He might have a multicolored bruise for up to ten days after donation. If he gets a bruise, apply ice for ten to fifteen minutes every half hour or so for the first day. After that, intermittently apply warm, moist heat to the area for ten to fifteen minutes.

Call the blood-donation center if:

☐ He gets a bruise larger than two or three inches in diameter

☐ He has redness, swelling, or pain at the needle-insertion area

☐ He experiences tingling in his fingers or arm

☐ He can't make the next appointment

Space for Your Notes:

....

....

These provisions appeared in my own living will. Use them as a checklist to make sure his reflects his wishes precisely.

☐ I direct my attending physicians to withhold or withdraw life-sustaining treatment that serves only to prolong the process of my dying, if I should be in a terminal condition.

☐ I also direct my attending physicians to withhold or withdraw life-sustaining treatment that serves only to prolong the process of my dying, if I should be in a state of permanent unconsciousness.

☐ I direct that treatment be limited to measures to keep me comfortable and to relieve pain, including any pain that might occur by withholding or withdrawing life-sustaining treatment.

☐ If I have a condition stated above, it is my preference not to receive tube feeding or any other artificial or invasive form of nutrition or hydration (food or water).

☐ In addition, if I have a condition stated above, I direct that the following forms of treatment be avoided:

☐ I do not want cardiac resuscitation.

☐ I do not want blood or blood products.

☐ I do not want mechanical respiration.

☐ I do not want antibiotics or other therapeutic medicines.

☐ I do not want dialysis.

☐ I do not want any surgery.

☐ I do not want any invasive procedures or tests.

☐ If I should be incompetent and in a condition stated above, I designate

_____,

currently residing at_____,

as my surrogate to make medical-treatment decisions for me. If he/she is unable to serve,

I designate _____,

currently residing at_____,

as my surrogate.

PREOPERATIVE EXAM CHECKLIST

Make sure he takes with him:

- ☐ Insurance cards
- ☐ General Medical History (pages 25–29; review it first)
- ☐ Copy of living will, advance directive, or health-care proxy
- ☐ List of questions
- ☐ List of dietary restrictions

If you plan to accompany him to the hospital, the following are questions you might wish to ask:

Where and when does he report? _____

What should he wear? _____

Anything else he should bring or leave at home? _____

How long will he be here? _____

Does his insurance cover everything?   ☐ Yes   ☐ No

If not, what is his responsibility? _____

Can he make special payment arrangements?   ☐ Yes   ☐ No   _____

How will I be advised of his condition? _____

After the operation, when can I see him?   ☐ Yes   ☐ No

When can family members visit? _____

Can grandchildren visit?   ☐ Yes   ☐ No   When? _____

Other questions:

....

....

....

....

....

....

....

....

....

....

....

LIST OF HEALTH-CARE PROVIDERS

Name	Position	How reached?

Space for Your Notes:

Resources

BOOKS AND BROCHURES ON PROSTATE CANCER

The American Cancer Society and the National Comprehensive Cancer Network, *Prostate Cancer: Treatment Guidelines for Patients*. Order a free copy at www.cancer.org or call (800) 227-2345.

Bostwick, David G., American Cancer Society, and Ron Schaumburg, *Prostate Cancer: What Every Man—and His Family—Needs to Know*. New York: Villard Books, 1999.

Korda, Michael, *Man to Man: Surviving Prostate Cancer*. New York: Vintage Books, 1997.

Lewis, James, Jr., *The Best Options for Diagnosing and Treating Prostate Cancer: Based on Research, Clinical Trials, and Scientific and Investigational Studies*. New York: Health Education Literary, 1994.

Lewis, James, Jr., with E. Roy Berger, *New Guidelines for Surviving Prostate Cancer*. New York: Health Education Literary, 1997.

Marks, Sheldon, *Prostate and Cancer: A Family Guide to Diagnosis, Treatment and Survival*. Tucson, AZ: Fisher Books, 2000.

Oesterling, Joseph A., and Mark A. Moyad, *The ABC's of Prostate Cancer: The Book That Could Save Your Life*. Lanham, MD: Madison Books, 1997.

Wainrib, Barbara Rubin, and Sandra Haber, *Men, Women, and Prostate Cancer*. Oakland, CA: New Harbinger Publications, 2000.

Walsh, Patrick C., *The Prostate: A Guide for Men and the Women Who Love Them*. New York: Warner Books, 1996.

GENERAL CANCER WEBSITES

Listed below are websites that contain information about cancer generally. (A few toll-free telephone numbers are listed as well.) Some of these sites offer links to prostate-cancer topics. A ton of material is included in these websites, so poke around and use your bookmarks liberally. If you do not have Internet access, do this research at your local library.

American Cancer Society
www.cancer.org
(800) 227-2345

National Cancer Institute
www.nci.nih.gov
(800) 4-CANCER

Oncology.com
Website: www.oncology.com

University of Pennsylvania
www.oncolink.upenn.edu

Cancer Care Inc.
www.cancercare.org
(800) 813-HOPE

National Library of Medicine
www.nlm.nih.gov

American Dietetic Association
www.eatright.org

United Kingdom Cancer-Help Site
www.cancerhelp.org.uk

For a comprehensive dictionary of medical terms, go to www.medicinenet.com and click on the "Dictionary" link.

PROSTATE-SPECIFIC WEBSITES

American Academy of Family Physicians
www.familydoctor.org/healthfacts/361

CaP Cure
www.capcure.org

Centerwatch Clinical-Trials Listing Service
www.centerwatch.com/patient/studies/CAT36.html

Department of Defense Center for Prostate-Disease Research
www.cpdr.org

Harvard Medical School Prostate Site
www.intelihealth.com/IH/ihtIH/WSIHW000/8294/8294.html

National Comprehensive Cancer Network
www.nccn.org

National Library of Health
(part of the National Institutes of Health)
www.nlm.nih.gov/medlineplus/prostatecancer.html

National Prostate-Cancer Coalition
www.4npcc.org

Phoenix5
www.phoenix5.org
Includes an excellent glossary of terms related to the disease.

Us Too!
www.ustoo.com

WEBSITES FOR CAREGIVERS

Helpful advice and resources for caregivers are available at the following Internet addresses:

The Cancer Survivors and Caregivers Network
www.acscsn.org

Family Caregiver Alliance
www.caregiver.org

National Family Caregivers Association
www.nfcacares.org

Caregiver Survival Resources
www.caregiver.com

Space for Your Notes:

Index

A

absorbent pads and briefs, 99
acupressure, 54
acupuncture, 54
advanced directives, 67
American Academy of Family
    Physicians, 138
American Board of Medical
    Specialties, 8
American Cancer Society, 137
American College of Surgeons, 127
American Dietetic Association, 137
American Medical Association, 8
American Red Cross, 62
antioxidants, 66
Association of Community Cancer
    Centers, 127
attending physician, 88

B

benign prostatic hyperplasia (BPH),
    6
biopsy, 13
blood donation, 62
body therapy, 55
bone scan, 32
brachytherapy, 43

C

caffeine, 65
Cancer Care Inc., 137
Cancer Hope Network, 80
cancer, stages of, 37; therapies for
    the treatment of, 42
Cancer Caregivers Network, 139

Cancer Survivors Network, 139
candy striper, 89
CaP Cure, 65, 138
caregivers, survival resources for,
    139; websites for, 139
catheter, 83; management and use
    of, 95; removal of, 97
Centerwatch Clinical Trials List, 108
chaplains, 90
chemical additives, 65
chemotherapy, 44
clinical trials, 108
computed tomography (CT Scan),
    32
consultant, 88

D

dental issues, 65
Department of Defense Center for
    Prostate-Disease Research, 138
depression, 76
diagnostic staff, 89
diet, issues relating to, 65
digital rectal exam (DRE), 6
Directory of Board Certified
    Medical Specialists, 8
Directory of Physicians in the
    United States, The, 8
driving, 93
durable health-care power of
    attorney, 67

E

erections, 102
exercise, 66
external radiation therapy, 42

F

family issues, 59
fellow, 88
follow-up, 107

G

Gleason scale, 15

H

Harvard Prostate Site, 138
health-care proxy, 67
herbal remedies, 53
home-care coordinators, 89
hormone therapy, 43
hospice staff, 90
hospital, food, 85; personnel, 88
hyperplasia, 6
hypnosis, 75

I

impotence, 102
incision, care of, 97
incontinence, 99
informed consent, 109
informing family, 59
intercourse alternatives, 105
intern, 88

J

journaling, 55

K

Kegel exercises, 98, 101

L

legal issues, 66
licensed practical nurses (LPNs),
    89
living will, 67

M

Man-to-Man, 80
massage, 55
medical history, 25
medical student, 88
meditation, 55

N

notekeeping, 1
National Cancer Institute, 127,
    137
National Cancer Network, 108
National Library of Health, 138
National Library of Medicine, 137
National Prostate Cancer
    Coalition, 138
nutritionist, 90

O

Oncology.com, 137
operating room, 82
orgasm, 102
"orange juice trick," 103

P

pain management, 93
partner, the role of a, 115
patient-care assistant (PCA), 89
patient-care technician (PCT), 89
patient rights and duties, 86
Patients Helping Patients, 80
penile implants, 104
penile injection, 104
penile suppository, 104
penis retraction, 95
Phoenix5, 80, 138
physicians assistant (PA), 89
post-op exercises, 84
pre-op examination, 71
prostate-specific antigen (PSA),
    13, 107
prostate, anatomy of, 5
prostatectomy, 44

Q

Quigong, 56

R

radical prostatectomy, 44
radiation therapy, 42
Red Cross, 62
registered nurse (RN), 89
relaxation response, 56
removal of catheter, 97
residents, 88
retraction of penis, 95

S

second opinions, 47
seeds (brachytherapy), 43
sensitive PSA, 107
sex issues, 70, 105
smoking, 65
social worker, 89
stages of cancer, 37
stress accidents, 100
student nurse, 89
suction pumps, 103
supplementary therapies, 53
support groups, 77, 80
surgery preparations, 71

T

Tai Chi, 57
tape recording, 2
therapies, 42
therapists, 90
transurethral prostatic resection
    (TURP), 7
treatment options, 42

U

ultrasound, 14
United Kingdom Cancer-Help
    site, 137
University of Pennsylvania
    Website, 137
urine bags, changing, 95
Us Too!, 80, 138

V

vacuum constriction device
    (VCD), 103
Viagra, 102
visiting nurses, 90, 96
vital statistics, 1
volatility of cells, 15

W

walking, 57, 92
watchful waiting, 42
websites, general cancer, 137;
    prostate-specific, 138
worksheets for partners, 116

X

X ray, 31

Y

Yoga, 57

THE CANCER PREVENTION BOOK: A Complete Mind/Body Approach to Stopping Cancer Before It Starts

by Rosy Daniel, M.D., with Rachel Ellis
Foreword by HRH the Prince of Wales

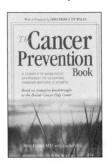

This guide to cancer prevention is based on the work of the world-famous Bristol Cancer Help Centre, one of the world's leading organizations specializing in holistic care for cancer patients. The key elements of this plan have helped thousands of cancer patients at the Centre, with many achieving remarkable recoveries. Dr Rosy Daniel guides readers step-by-step through identifying and removing risk factors from their lives to achieving high-energy health through the use of complementary therapies and nutritional regimens that build up the immune system and combat cancer. Specific subjetcs covered include anticancer foods and how they work; known and suspected carcinogens in household products and the environment; the effects of HRT and the Pill; and the importance of spiritual nourishment.

272 pages ... 14 charts ... Paperback $15.95 ... Hardcover $25.95

CANCER — INCREASING YOUR ODDS FOR SURVIVAL: A Resource Guide for Integrating Mainstream, Alternative and Complementary Therapies

by David Bognar, with a Preface by O. Carl Simonton, Ph.D.

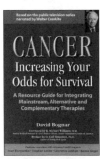

Based on the four-part television series hosted by Walter Cronkite.

Nothing increases a cancer patient's odds of survival more than quick access to the right information. From the first moment of diagnosis, patients need to know what questions to ask, how to evaluate treatments and where to go for additional help. This book describes all the current conventional, alternative, and complementary treatments for cancer. Each listing covers a treatment and its success rates and gives contact information for experts, organizations, and support groups as well as book, video, and Internet resource listings. Full-length interviews with leaders in the field of healing, including Joan Borysenko, Stephen Levine, and Bernie Siegel, cover the powerful effect the mind has on the body and the therapies that strengthen the connection between spiritual healing and issues of death and dying.

352 pages ... Paperback $15.95 ... Hardcover $25.95

MEN'S CANCERS: How to Prevent Them, How to Treat Them, How to Beat Them

by Pamela J. Haylock R.N., M.A., E.T., Editor

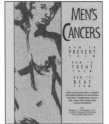

A complete resource for men diagnosed with or concerned about cancer. Each chapter, written by a specialized nurse or nurse practitioner, covers prevention, early detection, diagnosis, treatments, follow-up, and recurrence. Special chapters address sex changes related to cancer and future directions in research and study. An extensive resource section provides links to treatment centers, clinics, and support organizations.

368 pages ... 16 illus. ... Paperback $19.95 ... Hardcover $29.95

WOMEN'S CANCERS: How to Prevent Them, How to Treat Them, How to Beat Them

by Kerry A. McGinn, R.N., and Pamela J. Haylock, R.N. — Third edition coming in October 2002

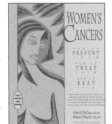

This guide gives women detailed information on treating and surviving the cancers that affect them: breast, cervical, ovarian, uterine, and vaginal cancer, as well as lung and colon cancer. The second edition covers latest screening guidelines, diagnostic tests, and the discovery of the breast cancer gene. The third edition will address late and long-term effects of cancer, new FDA approved and "smart" drugs; and possible environmental factors in cancer development.

2nd edition: 512 pages ... 68 illus. ... Paperback $19.95
3rd edition: 560 pages ... 72 illus. ... Paperback $24.95

CANCER DOESN'T HAVE TO HURT: How to Conquer the Pain Caused by Cancer and Cancer Treatment

by Pamela J. Haylock, R.N., M.A., and Carol P. Curtiss, R.N., OCN

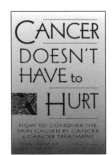

Leading the movement toward better pain control, Haylock and Curtiss show that cancer pain relief can be improved and patients who have less pain do better. Readers learn how to describe their pain clearly and to read prescriptions, administer medications, and adjust dosages if necessary. Also included are non-drug methods of pain relief, including massage, exercise, visual imagery, and music therapy.

192 pages ... 12 illus. ... Paperback $14.95 ... Hardcover $24.95

THE ART OF GETTING WELL: A Five-Step Plan for Maximizing Health When You Have a Chronic Illness

by David Spero, R.N., Foreword by Martin Rossman, M.D.

Self-management programs have become a key way for people to deal with chronic illness. In this book, Spero brings together the medical, psychological and spiritual aspects of getting well in a five-step approach that asks you to slow down and use your energy for the things that matter; make small, progressive changes that build confidence; get help and nourish the social ties that are crucial for well-being; value your body and treat it with affection and respect; and take responsibility for getting the best care you can.

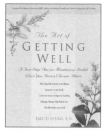

224 pages ... Paperback $15.95 ... Hardcover $25.95

CHINESE HERBAL MEDICINE MADE EASY: Natural and Effective Remedies for Common Illnesses

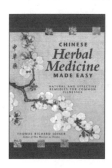

by Thomas Richard Joiner

Chinese herbal medicine is an ancient system for maintaining health and prolonging life. This book demystifies the subject, with clear explanations and alphabetical listings of 750 herbal remedies for over 250 common illnesses from acid reflux and AIDS to breast cancer, pain management, sexual dysfunction, and weight loss. Whether you are a newcomer to herbology or a seasoned practitioner, you will find this book a valuable addition to your health library.

400 pages ... Paperback $24.95 ... Hardcover $34.95

MAKING LOVE BETTER THAN EVER: Reaching New Heights of Passion and Pleasure After 40

by Barbara Keesling, Ph.D.

Great sex is not reserved for people under 40. With maturity comes the potential for a multi-faceted loving. In this book, Barbara Keesling shows how loving touch has the power to heighten sexual response and expand sexual potential; reduce anxiety and increase health and well-being; build self-esteem and improve body image; and promote playfulness, spontaneity, and a natural sense of joy.

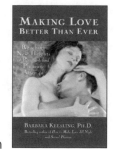

208 pages ... 14 b/w photos ... Paperback $13.95

POSITIVE OPTIONS FOR LIVING WITH YOUR OSTOMY: Self-Help and Treatment

Dr. Craig A. White

An ostomy is a surgically created opening used to expel waste when the body's normal systems are damaged. This book helps you to deal with the practical and emotional aspects of life after ostomy surgery. It describes what happens in the surgery; how to adapt to wearing ostomy care appliances, and how to care for and change them. It provides information on dealing with emotional reactions, including anxiety and depression, and knowing when to seek help. Helpful lists provide structures for dealing with changes in social relationships and sexual activity.

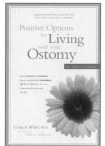

144 pages ... Paperback $12.95 ... Hardcover $22.95

POSITIVE OPTIONS FOR CROHN'S DISEASE: Self-Help and Treatment

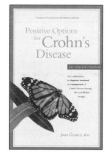

by Joan Gomez, M.D.

Crohn's disease is an inflammatory bowel condition that, while non-fatal, can be devastating. This book discusses who is at risk and why and outlines the most up-to-date treatments available, including natural and prescription medications and effective surgical options, with detailed advice about life (including sex) after surgery. Self-care options, in which dietary changes are key, are described in detail, from constructing a personal diet plan to boosting the immune system through nutrition and special diets.

192 pp. ... 1 b/w illus. ... Paperback $12.95

POSITIVE OPTIONS FOR HIATUS HERNIA: Self-Help and Treatment

by Tom Smith, M.D.

Do you have frequent heartburn or acid reflux? Do you take antacids by the handful and worry that you have an ulcer? You may have a hiatus hernia. This book describes how this condition happens and how to protect yourself from serious consequences like esophageal cancer. It includes the latest tests and medical treatments, drug and surgery options, and self-help options for diet, eating habits, and stress management.

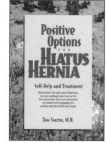

160 pp. ... 12 b/w illus. ... Paperback $12.95 ... Hardcover $22.95

Prices subject to change ... for latest information please call 1-800-266-5592

ORDER FORM

10%	DISCOUNT on orders of $50 or more —	
20%	DISCOUNT on orders of $150 or more —	
30%	DISCOUNT on orders of $500 or more —	

On cost of books for fully prepaid orders

NAME

ADDRESS

CITY/STATE   ZIP/POSTCODE

PHONE   COUNTRY (outside of U.S.)

TITLE	QTY	PRICE	TOTAL
Prostate Health Workbook (paperback)		@ $14.95	
Prostate Health Workbook (hardcover)		@ $24.95	

Prices subject to change without notice

Please list other titles below:

		@ $	
		@ $	
		@ $	
		@ $	
		@ $	
		@ $	
		@ $	

Check here to receive our book catalog   ❏   FREE

Shipping Costs:
*First book: $4.00 by book post ($5.00 by UPS, Priority Mail, or to ship outside the U.S.)
Each additional book: $1.00
For rush orders and bulk shipments call us at (800) 266-5592*

TOTAL	_____
Less discount @_____%	(_____)
TOTAL COST OF BOOKS	_____
Calif. residents add sales tax	_____
Shipping & handling	_____
TOTAL ENCLOSED	_____

Please pay in U.S. funds only

❏ Check ❏ Money Order ❏ Visa ❏ MasterCard ❏ Discover

Card # _____   Exp. date _____

Signature _____

Complete and mail to:
Hunter House Inc., Publishers
PO Box 2914, Alameda CA 94501-0914
Phone (510) 865-5282 Fax (510) 865-4295
Ordering: (800) 266-5592 / ordering@hunterhouse.com
website: www.hunterhouse.com

PWB — April 2002